Immediate Life Support

4th Edition January 2016

Reprinted in August 2016
Reprinted in March 2017
Reprinted in March 2018

ISBN 978-1-903812-31-0

ILS

Immediate Life Support

4th Edition January 2016 – Reprinted in August 2016 / March 2017 / March 2018

Editors

Jasmeet Soar

Jerry Nolan

Sue Hampshire

Sarah Mitchell

Contributors

Matthew Cordingly

Ron Daniels

Robin Davies

Charles Deakin

James Fullerton

David Gabbott

Carl Gwinnutt

Sue Hampshire

Andrew Lockey

Kevin Mackie

Oliver Meyer

Sarah Mitchell

Jerry Nolan

Gavin Perkins

David Pitcher

Susanna Price

Mike Scott

Gary Smith

Jasmeet Soar

Joyce Yeung

Acknowledgements

We thank Mike Scott for taking and digitally preparing all the photographs in this manual. We also thank the Nuffield Hospital, Guildford, for the use of their facilities, Oliver Meyer for digital preparation of the rhythm strips, Paul Wood at TT Litho Printers Limited for help with the final preparation for printing, and the models who gave up their time to help with the photographs.

Printed on responsibly sourced environmentally friendly paper made with elemental chlorine free fibre from legal and sustainably managed forests.

Chain of Prevention © Gary Smith

ECGs © Oliver Meyer

Electrical conduction of the heart (Figure 6.3) © LifeART image (1989-2001) Wolters Kluwer Health, Inc.-Lippincott Williams & Wilkins. All rights reserved.

Photographs © Mike Scott

Published by Resuscitation Council (UK)
5th Floor, Tavistock House North, Tavistock Square, London WC1H 9HR
Tel: 020 7388 4678   Fax: 020 7383 0773   E-mail: enquiries@resus.org.uk   Website: www.resus.org.uk

Printed by: All About Print
Tel: 020 7205 4022   Email: hello@allaboutprint.co.uk   Website: www.allaboutprint.co.uk

The Resuscitation Council (UK) guidelines are adapted from the European Resuscitation Council guidelines and have been developed using a process accredited by The National Institute for Health and Care Excellence. The UK guidelines are consistent with the European guidelines but include minor modifications to reflect the needs of the National Health Service.

This Immediate Life Support manual forms part of the resources for the Resuscitation Council (UK) course, which is delivered in accredited course centres throughout the UK.

Immediate Life Support

ILS

The Resuscitation Council (UK) Immediate Life Support (ILS) course provides you with essential knowledge and skills to treat adults with cardiorespiratory arrest for the short time before the arrival of a resuscitation team or more experienced help. It also prepares you to help the resuscitation team.

Many cardiorespiratory arrests are preventable and ILS teaches the recognition and treatment of the deteriorating patient using the ABCDE (Airway, Breathing, Circulation, Disability, Exposure) approach. ILS knowledge and skills will help you recognise and start treating the deteriorating patient. If cardiorespiratory arrest does occur, the skills taught on the ILS course are those that are most likely to resuscitate the patient.

The Chain of Survival describes the interventions that contribute to patient survival. The ILS course teaches the important knowledge and skills for each link in the chain. The strength of the whole chain is dependent on the strength of each of the four links . They are:

- Early recognition and call for help – to prevent cardiac arrest

- Early cardiopulmonary resuscitation (CPR) – to buy time

- Early defibrillation – to restart the heart

- Post-resuscitation care – to restore quality of life

The knowledge presented in this manual is predominantly about the resuscitation of patients in an acute hospital;

however, the initial resuscitation of patients is similar in any clinical setting (e.g. community hospital). The same core standards apply to all clinical settings. These are:

- The deteriorating patient is recognised early and there is an effective system to summon help in order to prevent cardiorespiratory arrest.

- Cardiorespiratory arrest is recognised early and cardiopulmonary resuscitation (CPR) is started immediately.

- Emergency assistance is summoned immediately, as soon as cardiorespiratory arrest is recognised, if help has not been summoned already.

- Defibrillation, if appropriate, is attempted within 3 minutes of identifying cardiorespiratory arrest.

- Post-cardiac arrest care is received by those who are resuscitated successfully. This includes safe transfer.

- Implementation of standards is measured continually and processes are in place to deal with any problems identified.

- Staff receive at least annual training and updates in CPR, based on their expected roles.

- Staff have an understanding of decisions relating to CPR.

- Appropriate equipment is immediately available for resuscitation.

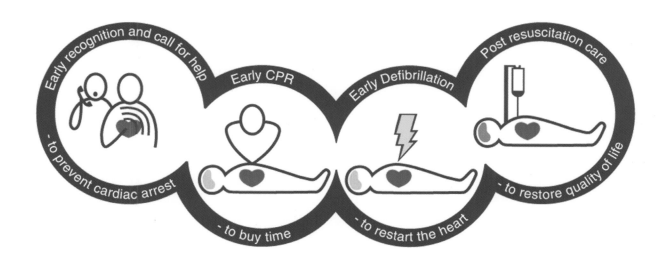

Glossary

- The masculine pronouns he, him, and his are used generically

- ABCDE refers to the Airway, Breathing, Circulation, Disability, Exposure approach

- AED is an automated external defibrillator

- CPR is cardiopulmonary resuscitation – this refers to chest compressions and ventilations

- ECG is electrocardiogram

- IV is intravenous

- IO is intraosseous – this refers to infusion of drugs or fluids into the bone marrow through a special needle inserted into a bone

- PEA is pulseless electrical activity

- ROSC is return of spontaneous circulation

- SBAR is a communication tool – Situation, Background, Assessment, Recommendation

- Shockable rhythm refers to cardiac arrest rhythms that can be treated with CPR and a defibrillator

- VF is ventricular fibrillation – VF is a shockable cardiac arrest rhythm

- VT is ventricular tachycardia

- pVT is pulseless ventricular tachycardia – pVT is a shockable cardiac arrest rhythm

- VF/pVT means VF or pulseless VT – these are both shockable cardiac arrest rhythms

Contents

Improving patient outcomes from cardiac arrest and deterioration

Chapter 1

Contents

- **Evidence based guidelines**
- **Quality standards**
- **Measuring patient outcomes**
- **Safety-incident reporting**
- **Non-technical skills**
- **Use of communications tools**

Learning outcomes

To enable you to:

- **Understand the importance of measuring patient outcomes and safety incident reporting to improve care**
- **Be an effective team member**
- **Consider the role of non-technical skills during resuscitation**
- **Effectively use structured communication tools such as SBAR and RSVP**

Introduction

High quality care is safe, effective, patient-centered, timely, efficient and equitable. Hospitals, resuscitation teams and ILS providers should ensure they deliver these aspects of quality to improve the care and outcomes of deteriorating patients and patients in cardiac arrest. Interventions to improve patient outcomes are described below and include:

- the use of evidence based guidelines

- quality standards

- measuring patient outcomes

- safety-incident reporting

- non-technical skills

- use of communications tools.

Evidence based guidelines

Improving outcomes from cardiac arrest depends on the implementation of evidence based guidelines. Immediate Life Support is consistent with the current Resuscitation Council (UK) Guidelines. The process used to produce these guidelines has been accredited by the National Institute for Health and Care Excellence. The guidelines are based on:

- Systematic reviews with grading of the quality of evidence and strength of recommendations.

- The involvement of stakeholders including members of the public and cardiac arrest survivors so that their values and preferences can be considered in guidelines.

The current Resuscitation Council (UK) Guidelines for cardiopulmonary resuscitation can be found at (www.resus.org.uk).

Quality standards

Hospitals and health care settings are obliged to provide a high quality resuscitation service that ensures staff are trained according to their expected roles. The same core standards apply to all healthcare settings to ensure that:

- The deteriorating patient is recognised early and there is an effective system to summon help in order to prevent cardiorespiratory arrest.

- Cardiorespiratory arrest is recognised early and cardiopulmonary resuscitation (CPR) is started immediately.

- Emergency assistance is summoned immediately, as soon as cardiorespiratory arrest is recognised, if help has not been summoned already.

- Defibrillation, if appropriate, is attempted within 3 minutes of identifying cardiorespiratory arrest.

- Appropriate post-cardiorespiratory-arrest care is received by those who are resuscitated successfully. This includes safe transfer.

- Implementation of standards is measured continually and processes are in place to deal with any problems identified.

- Staff receive at least annual training and updates in CPR, based on their expected roles.

- Staff have an understanding of decisions relating to CPR.

- Appropriate equipment is immediately available for resuscitation.

The Resuscitation Council (UK) *Quality standards for cardiopulmonary resuscitation practice and training* provide further detailed information. These standards include suggested equipment lists for different health care settings.

Measuring patient outcomes

Continuous measurement of compliance with processes, and patient outcomes at a national and local level provides information on the impact of changes in practice, identifies areas for improvement, and also enables comparison in outcomes between different organisations. There are uniform definitions for collecting data for cardiac arrest.

The National Cardiac Arrest Audit (NCAA) is an ongoing, national, comparative outcome audit of in-hospital cardiac arrests. It is a joint initiative between the Resuscitation

Council (UK) and the Intensive Care National Audit & Research Centre (ICNARC) and is open to all acute hospitals in the UK and Ireland. The audit monitors and reports on the incidence of, and outcome from, in-hospital cardiac arrest in order to inform practice and policy. Data are collected on individuals receiving chest compressions and/or defibrillation who are attended by the hospital resuscitation team in response to a 2222 call. Data are collected according to standardised definitions and entered onto the NCAA secure web-based system. Once data are validated, hospitals are provided with activity reports and risk-adjusted comparative reports, allowing a comparison to be made not only within, but also between, hospitals locally, nationally and internationally. Recent data from 144 hospitals showed the overall incidence of adult in-hospital cardiac arrest was 1.6 per 1000 hospital admissions, and varied seasonally, peaking in winter. The overall survival to hospital discharge was 18.4%.

The National Out of Hospital Cardiac Arrest Outcomes project measures patient, process and outcome variables from out-of-hospital-cardiac arrest in the UK. The project is run in collaboration with the National Ambulance Service Medical Directors Group with support from the British Heart Foundation, the Resuscitation Council (UK) and the University of Warwick. The project is designed to measure the epidemiology, and outcomes of cardiac arrest and to serve as a national resource for continuous quality improvement initiatives for cardiac arrest.

Safety incident reporting

In England and Wales, hospitals can report patient safety incidents to the National Reporting and Learning System (NRLS) (http://www.nrls.npsa.nhs.uk/report-a-patient-safety-incident/). A patient safety incident is defined as 'any unintended or unexpected incident that could have harmed or did lead to harm for one or more patients being cared for by the National Health Service (NHS)'. Resuscitation related incidents are associated with equipment problems, communication, delays in the resuscitation team attending, and failure to escalate treatment.

Non-technical skills

Chest compressions and defibrillation are considered as the most important factors in managing a cardiac arrest. These are both technical skills that you can learn from books, lectures, courses and colleagues. Although these are important for successful resuscitation, there is another group of skills that are now recognised as being equally important – non-technical skills. Non-technical skills are the cognitive, social and personal resource skills that together with technical skills help deliver safe and effective care to patients. More simply, non-technical skills are the things that affect your personal performance.

The importance of non-technical skills in emergencies is now widely accepted. Examples of poor non-technical skills leading to system errors and worse patient outcomes after cardiac arrest include:

- unwillingness to help

- poor communication

- a lack of clear roles and responsibilities.

Understanding and improving non-technical skills may help to reduce human errors, creating more effective teams and improve patient outcomes. Non-technical skills include:

- situational awareness

- decision making

- team working, including team leadership

- task management.

Situational awareness

This is your awareness of what is happening during an event and your understanding of how what you do will change things. This is important when many events are happening at the same time such as at a cardiac arrest. At a cardiac arrest, team members often have varying degrees of situational awareness. In a well-functioning team, all members will have shared situational awareness – everybody knows what is happening and is working to the same game plan. It is important that only the relevant information is shared otherwise there is too much distraction and noise.

To improve situational awareness at a cardiac arrest:

- consider the location of the arrest for clues to the cause

- obtain information about the events leading up to the arrest

- confirm the diagnosis

- determine who is present – including names, roles, and who is leading

- note actions already started (e.g. chest compressions)

- communicate with other team members and gather information

- implement any immediate action necessary (e.g. start chest compressions)

- consider the likely impact of interventions

- determine immediate needs (e.g. need for suction).

Decision making

This is choosing a specific plan of action from several alternatives. At a cardiac arrest, decision making usually falls to the most senior clinician present (e.g. nurse, or junior doctor, until more senior help arrives). This person will need to take on a leadership role before the resuscitation team arrives. The leader will assimilate information from those present and from personal

observation and will use this to determine appropriate interventions. Typical immediate decisions made at a cardiac arrest include:

- confirmation of cardiac arrest

- calling the resuscitation team

- starting CPR

- attaching a defibrillator and delivering a shock.

Once a decision has been made, clear unambiguous communication is essential to ensure that it is implemented. For example, a nurse finding a patient in cardiac arrest asks her colleague to call the resuscitation team – "*John, this man has had a cardiac arrest. Please dial 2222 and call the resuscitation team. Come back with the resuscitation trolley when you have done this*".

Team working, including team leadership

This is one of the most important non-technical skills in an emergency. A team is a group of individuals working together with a common goal or purpose. In a team, members usually have complementary skills and with a joint effort you will achieve more than if you work alone. Teams work best when:

- Everyone knows each other's name.

- The team is doing something they think is important.

- Team members are working within their experience and competence.

To be a good resuscitation team member you will be:

- Competent in the skills required at a cardiac arrest and perform them to the best of your ability and according to your expected role.

- Committed to achieve the best outcome for the patient.

- Able to communicate openly, indicating your findings and actions.

- Prepared to raise concerns about clinical or safety issues, and also listen to briefings and instructions from the team leader.

- Supportive, enabling others to achieve their best.

- Accountable for your own and the team's actions.

- Prepared to admit when help is needed.

- Creative suggesting different ways of interpreting the situation.

- Involved in providing feedback.

Team leadership

The team leader provides guidance, direction and instruction to the team members to enable successful completion of their stated objective (Figure 1.1). They lead by example and integrity. Team leaders need experience not simply seniority. Team leadership can be considered a process; it is available to everyone with training and is not restricted to those with leadership traits. To be a good team leader you need to:

- Know everyone in the team by name and know their capability.

- Accept the leadership role.

- Delegate tasks appropriately.

- Be knowledgeable and credible to influence the team through role modelling and professionalism.

- Stay calm and keep everyone focused and control distractions.

- Communicate – do not just give orders, but be a good listener and be decisive.

- Show empathy towards the team.

- Be assertive and authoritative when required.

- Tolerate hesitancy or nervousness in the emergency setting and be supportive.

- Have good situational awareness; constantly monitor the situation, with an up-to-date overview, listen and decide on a course of action.

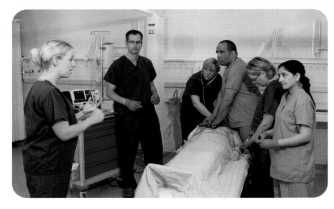

Figure 1.1 Team leadership

Those doing the Resuscitation Council (UK) ILS course are not expected to be resuscitation team leaders. You may have to take a lead role before the team arrives however. During a cardiac arrest, the role of team leader is not always immediately obvious. The leader should state early on that they are assuming the role of team leader. At a cardiac arrest the leader should:

- Follow current resuscitation guidelines or explain the reason for not doing so.

- If unsure, ask the team or call for senior advice and assistance.

- Play to the strengths of team members and allow them some autonomy if their skills are adequate.

- Allocate roles and tasks throughout the resuscitation and be specific. This avoids several people or nobody attempting the task!

- Use the 2-minute periods of chest compressions to plan tasks and safety aspects of the resuscitation attempt with the team.

- Thank the team at the end of the resuscitation attempt and ensure that staff and relatives are being supported.

- Complete all documentation and ensure an adequate handover.

Task management

During the resuscitation of a deteriorating or cardiac arrest patient, team members do numerous tasks either sequentially or simultaneously. The coordination and control of these tasks is the responsibility of the team leader (Figure 1.2). They include:

- Planning, where appropriate, and briefing the team, prior to the arrival of the patient.

- Being inclusive of team members.

- Being prepared for both the expected and the unexpected.

- Identifying resources required – ensuring that equipment is checked and specifics organised and delegated.

- Prioritising actions of the team.

- Watching out for fatigue, stress and distress amongst the team.

- Managing conflict.

- Communicating with relatives.

- Communicating with experts for safe handover both by telephone and in person.

- Debriefing the team.

- Reporting untoward incidents, particularly equipment or system failures.

- Participating in audit.

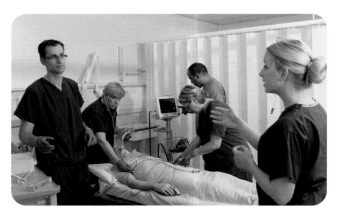

Figure 1.2 Task management

The importance of communication when managing a deteriorating patient

Communication problems contribute to 80% of adverse incidents or near miss reports in hospitals. This failure of communication is also evident when a medical emergency occurs on a ward and a doctor or nurse asks for senior help. The call for help is often suboptimal, with failure by the caller to convey information in a way that informs the recipient of the urgency of the situation. A well-structured process that is simple, reliable and dependable, will enable the caller to convey the important facts and urgency, and will help the recipient to plan ahead.

The use of the SBAR (Situation, Background, Assessment, Recommendation) or RSVP (Reason, Story, Vital signs, Plan) tool enables effective, timely communication between individuals from different clinical backgrounds and hierarchies (Table 1.1). Learn and use the system that is used in your hospital.

Resuscitation teams

The resuscitation team may take the form of a traditional cardiac arrest team, which is called only when cardiac arrest is recognised. Alternatively, many hospitals now have strategies to recognise patients at risk of cardiac arrest and call a team (e.g. medical emergency team) before cardiac arrest occurs (Chapter 2). The term resuscitation team reflects the range of response teams. As the team may change daily or more frequently, as shift pattern working is introduced, members may not know each other or the skill mix of the team members. Team members should therefore meet at the beginning of their period on duty (Figure 1.3) to:

- Introduce themselves to each other; communication is much easier and more effective if people are referred to by their name. It is much harder to speak up or voice a concern in the absence of a modest degree of familiarity.

- Identify everyone's skills and experience.

- Allocate the team leader. Skill and experience takes precedence over seniority.

- Allocate responsibilities; if key skills are lacking (e.g. nobody skilled in advanced airway management) work out how this deficit can be managed.

- Review any patients who have been identified as 'at risk' during the previous duty period.

Ward staff can also plan roles and responsibilities for dealing with an emergency at the start of each shift.

Finally, every effort should be made to enable the team members to debrief. An immediate post-event debriefing ('Hot' debriefing) is normally led by the resuscitation team leader, focuses on immediate issues and concerns, and is

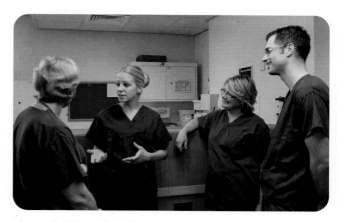

Figure 1.3 Team briefing

usually of short duration. This can be difficult if the patient has a return of spontaneous circulation, as focus then inevitably shifts to post-resuscitation care.

A delayed facilitated debriefing ('Cold' debriefing) can also be useful.

Summary learning

- **Report safety incidents and collect cardiac arrest data to help improve patient care.**
- **Non-technical skills are very important during resuscitation.**
- **Use SBAR or RSVP for effective communication.**

My key take-home messages from this chapter

SBAR	RSVP	Content	Example

SITUATION	**R**EASON	• Introduce yourself and check you are speaking to the correct person
		
		• Identify the patient you are calling about (who and where)
		
		• Say what you think the current problem is, or appears to be
		
		• State what you need advice about
		
		• Useful phrases:
		
		  - The problem appears to be cardiac/respiratory/neurological/sepsis
		
		  - I'm not sure what the problem is but the patient is deteriorating
		
		  - The patient is unstable, getting worse and I need help
			• Hi, I'm John, staff nurse on the acute medical admission ward
			
			• I am calling about Mr Brown who was admitted with severe pneumonia
			
			• He has an oxygen saturation of 90% despite high-flow oxygen and I am very worried about him

BACKGROUND	**S**TORY	• Background information about the patient • Reason for admission • Relevant past medical history	• He is 55 and previously fit and well • He has had fever and a cough for 2 days • He arrived one hour ago by ambulance
ASSESSMENT	**V**ITAL SIGNS	• Include specific observations and vital sign values based on ABCDE approach • Airway • Breathing • Circulation • Disability • Exposure • The early warning score is...	• He looks very unwell and is tiring • Airway – he can say a few words • Breathing – his respiratory rate is 24. His oxygen saturation is 90% on high-flow oxygen • Circulation – his pulse is 110, his blood pressure is 110/60 • Disability – he is drowsy but can say a few words. He is confused • Exposure – he is pale and clammy • His early warning score is....

RECOMMENDATION	**P**LAN	• State explicitly what you want the person you are calling to do
		
		• What by when?
		
		• Useful phrases:
		
		  - I am going to start the following treatment; is there anything else you can suggest?
		
		  - I am going to do the following investigations; is there anything else you can suggest?
		
		  - If they do not improve; when would you like to be called?
		
		  - I don't think I can do any more; I would like you to see the patient urgently
			• I have given him the IV antibiotics that you prescribed and he has had 1 litre of IV saline
			
			• I am worried he is getting worse. I need help – please can you come and see him straight away

Table 1.1 SBAR and RSVP communication tools

Further reading

Andersen PO, Jensen MK, Lippert A, et al: Identifying non-technical skills and barriers for improvement of teamwork in cardiac arrest teams. Resuscitation 2010; 81:695–702.

Featherstone P, Chalmers T, Smith GB. RSVP: a system for communication of deterioration in hospital patients. Br J Nurs 2008;17: 860-64.

Flin R, O'Connor P, Crichton M. Safety at the Sharp End: a Guide to Non-Technical Skills. Aldershot: Ashgate, 2008.

National Out of Hospital Cardiac Arrest Outcomes Project. www.warwick.ac.uk/ohcao

Nolan JP, Hazinski MF, Aicken R, et al. Part I. Executive Summary: 2015 International Consensus on cardiopulmonary Resuscitation and Emergency Cardiovascular Care Science with Treatment Recommendations. Resuscitation 2015;95:e1-e32.

Nolan JP, Soar J, Smith GB, et al. Incidence and outcome of in-hospital cardiac arrest in the United Kingdom National Cardiac Arrest Audit. Resuscitation 2014;85:987-92.

Perkins GD, Handley AJ, Koster KW, et al. European Resuscitation Council Guidelines for Resuscitation 2015 Section 2 Adult basic life support and automated external defibrillation. Resuscitation 2015;95:81-98.

Resuscitation Council (UK). Quality standards for cardiopulmonary resuscitation and training. https://www.resus.org.uk/quality-standards/

Soar J, Callaway CW, Aibiki M, et al. Part 4: Advanced life support: 2015 International Consensus on Cardiopulmonary Resuscitation and Emergency Cardiovascular Care Science With Treatment Recommendations. Resuscitation 2015;95:e71-e122.

Soar J, Nolan JP, Bottiger BW, et al. European Resuscitation Council Guidelines for Resuscitation 2015 Section 3 Adult Advanced Life Support. Resuscitation 2015;95:99-146.

United Kingdom National Cardiac Arrest Audit. https://www.icnarc.org/Our-Audit/Audits/Ncaa/About

Yeung J, Ong G, Davies R, Gao F, Perkins GDP. Factors affecting team leadership skills and their relationship with quality of cardiopulmonary resuscitation. Crit Care Med 2012;40:2617–2621.

ILS

Recognising deterioration and preventing cardiorespiratory arrest

Contents

- **Prevention of in-hospital cardiac arrest: the Chain of Prevention**
- **Recognising the deteriorating patient**
- **Response to critical illness**
- **Causes of deterioration and cardiorespiratory arrest**
- **The ABCDE approach**

Learning outcomes

To enable you to:

- **Understand the importance of early recognition of the deteriorating patient**
- **Consider the relevant causes of cardiorespiratory arrest in adults**
- **Identify and treat patients at risk of cardiorespiratory arrest using the Airway, Breathing, Circulation, Disability, Exposure (ABCDE) approach**

Introduction

Early recognition of the deteriorating patient and prevention of cardiac arrest is the first link in the Chain of Survival. Once cardiac arrest occurs, about 20% of patients having an in-hospital cardiac arrest survive to go home. Prevention of in-hospital cardiac arrest requires staff education, monitoring of patients, recognition of patient deterioration, a system to call for help, and an effective response.

Survivors from in-hospital cardiac arrest usually have a witnessed and monitored ventricular fibrillation (VF) arrest, primary myocardial ischaemia as the cause, and receive immediate and successful defibrillation (e.g. on the coronary care unit).

Most in-hospital cardiac arrests are not sudden or unpredictable events: in up to 80% of cases there is deterioration in clinical signs during the few hours before cardiac arrest. These patients often have slow and progressive physiological deterioration, particularly hypoxia and hypotension (i.e. Airway, Breathing, Circulation problems) that is unnoticed by staff, or is recognised but treated poorly. The cardiac arrest rhythm in this group is usually non-shockable (pulseless electrical activity (PEA) or asystole) and very few patients survive and leave hospital.

Early recognition and effective treatment of the deteriorating patient might prevent cardiac arrest, death or an unanticipated intensive care unit (ICU) admission. Early recognition will also help to identify individuals for whom cardiopulmonary resuscitation (CPR) is not appropriate or who do not wish to be resuscitated (Chapter 10).

Much of this chapter is based on the deteriorating patient in the hospital setting. The same basic principles however apply to the care of the deteriorating patient in the out-of-hospital setting.

Prevention of in-hospital cardiac arrest: the Chain of Prevention

The Chain of Prevention (Figure 2.1) can assist hospitals in structuring care processes to prevent and detect patient deterioration and cardiac arrest. The five rings of the chain represent:

- **Education:** how to observe patients; interpretation of observed signs; the recognition of signs of deterioration; the use of the ABCDE approach; simple skills to stabilise the patient pending the arrival of more experienced help; knowledge of rationale for and role in the rapid response system in use in the hospital.

- **Monitoring:** patient assessment and the measurement and recording of vital signs, which may include the use of electronic monitoring and/or documentation devices.

- **Recognition** encompasses the tools available to identify patients in need of additional monitoring or intervention, including suitably designed vital signs charts and sets of predetermined 'calling criteria' to 'flag' the need to escalate monitoring or to call for more expert help.

- **Call for help** protocols for summoning a response to a deteriorating patient should be universally known and understood, unambiguous and mandated. Doctors and nurses often find it difficult to ask for help or escalate treatment as they feel their clinical judgement may be criticised. Hospitals should ensure all staff are empowered to call for help. Call for help by using a structured communication tool such as SBAR (Situation, Background, Assessment, Recommendation) or RSVP (Reason, Story, Vital signs, Plan).

- **Response** to a deteriorating patient must be assured, of specified speed and by staff with appropriate acute or critical care skills and experience (e.g. from the outreach or intensive care unit team).

Recognising the deteriorating patient

In general, the clinical signs of critical illness are similar whatever the underlying process because they reflect failing respiratory, cardiovascular, and neurological systems (i.e. ABCDE problems) (see below). It is common for ward patients to have abnormal vital signs, but vital sign observations are not done as often as they should be, especially at night.

To help early detection of deteriorating patients, many hospitals use early warning scores (EWS). The score of one or more vital sign observations, or the total EWS, indicates the level of intervention required (e.g. increased frequency of vital signs monitoring, or calling ward doctors or resuscitation teams to the patient).In the UK, the National Early Warning Score is recommended (Table 2.1).

Early warning scores are dynamic and change over time and the frequency of observations should be increased to track improvement or deterioration in a patient's condition. If it is clear a patient is deteriorating call for help early rather than waiting for the patient to reach a specific score.

The patient's EWS is calculated based on Table 2.1. An increased score indicates an increased risk of deterioration and death. There should be a graded response to scores according to local hospital protocols. An example escalation plan is shown in Table 2.2.

Alternatively, systems incorporating calling criteria are based on routine observations, which activate a response when one or more variables reach an extremely abnormal value. Recent research suggests that EWS may be better discriminators of outcomes than calling criteria. Some hospitals combine elements of both systems.

Nurse concern may also be an important predictor of patient deterioration. Even when doctors are alerted to a patient's abnormal physiology, there is often delay in attending to the patient or referring to higher levels of care.

Response to critical illness

The traditional response to cardiac arrest is reactive: the name 'cardiac arrest team' implies that it will be called only after cardiac arrest has occurred. In many hospitals, the cardiac arrest team has been replaced by other teams (e.g. rapid response team, critical care outreach team,

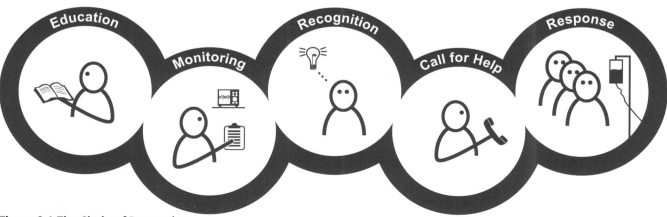

Figure 2.1 The Chain of Prevention

Physiological parameter		Score 3	2	1	0	1	2	3
A & B	Respiration rate (per minute)	≤8		9–11	12–20		21–24	≥25
	SpO$_2$ Scale 1 (%)	≤91	92–93	94–95	≥96			
	SpO$_2$ Scale 2 (%)*	≤83	84–85	86–87	88–92 ≥93 on air	93–94 on oxygen	95–96 on oxygen	≥97 on oxygen
	Air or oxygen?		Oxygen		Air			
C	Systolic blood pressure (mmHg)	≤90	91–100	101–110	111–219			≥220
	Pulse (per minute)	≤40		41–50	51–90	91–110	111–130	≥131
D	Consciousness**				Alert			Confusion VPU
E	Temperature (°C)	≤35.0		35.1–36.0	36.1–38.0	38.1–39.0	≥39.1	

* Use Scale 2 if target range is 88–92% (e.g. in hypercapnic respiratory failure).

** Score for new onset confusion, no score if chronic confusion.

Table 2.1 National Early Warning Score

medical emergency team (MET)). These teams can be activated according to the patient's EWS (see above) or according to specific calling criteria. For example, the MET usually comprises medical and nursing staff from intensive care and acute medicine and responds to specific calling criteria and cardiac arrests. Any member of the healthcare team, and in some cases the patient or their relatives, can initiate a MET call. Early involvement of the MET may reduce cardiac arrests, deaths and unanticipated ICU admissions, and may facilitate decisions about limitation of treatment (e.g. do not attempt resuscitation CPR (DNACPR) decisions). Medical emergency team interventions often involve simple tasks such as starting oxygen therapy and intravenous fluids. The benefits of the MET system remain to be proved, but evidence of their worth is increasing.

In the UK, a system of pre-emptive ward care known as critical care outreach, has developed. Outreach services exist in many forms ranging from a single nurse to a 24-hour, seven days per week multiprofessional team. An outreach team or system may reduce ward deaths, postoperative adverse events, ICU admissions and readmissions, and increase survival. Rapid response teams, such as outreach teams or METs, play a role in educating and improving acute care skills of ward personnel.

Critically ill patients should be admitted to a critical care area (e.g. ICU, high dependency unit (HDU), or resuscitation room). These areas are staffed by doctors and nurses experienced in advanced resuscitation and critical care skills.

Hospital staffing tends to be at its lowest during the night and at weekends. This influences patient monitoring, treatment and outcomes. In-hospital cardiac arrests occurring in the late afternoon, at night or at weekends are more often non-witnessed and have a lower survival rate. Patients discharged at night from ICUs to general wards have an increased risk of ICU readmission and in-hospital death compared with those discharged during the day and those discharged to HDUs.

Causes of deterioration and cardiorespiratory arrest

Deterioration and cardiorespiratory arrest can be caused by airway and/or breathing and/or cardiovascular problems.

NEW score	Frequency of monitoring	Clinical response
0	Minimum 12 hourly	• Continue routine NEWS monitoring.
Total 1-4	Minimum 4-6 hourly	• Inform registered nurse, who must assess the patient. • Registered nurse decides whether increased frequency of monitoring and/or escalation of care is required.
3 in single parameter	Minimum 1 hourly	• Registered nurse to inform medical team caring for the patient, who will review and decide whether escalation of care is necessary.
Total 5 or 6 Urgent response threshold	Minimum 1 hourly	• Registered nurse to immediately inform the medical team caring for the patient. • Registered nurse to request urgent assessment by a clinician or team with core competencies in the care of acutely ill patients. • Provide clinical care in an environment with monitoring facilities.
Total 7 or more Emergency response threshold	Continuous monitoring of vital signs	• Registered nurse to immediately inform the medical team caring for the patient – this should be at least at specialist registrar level. • Emergency assessment by a team with critical care competencies, including practitioner(s) with advanced airway management skills. • Consider transfer of care to a level 2 or 3 clinical care facility i.e. higher-dependency unit or ICU. • Clinical care in an environment with monitoring facilities.

Table 2.2 Escalation protocol based on early warning score

Airway obstruction

For a detailed review of airway management see Chapter 5.

Causes of airway obstruction

Airway obstruction can be complete or partial. Complete airway obstruction rapidly causes cardiac arrest. Partial obstruction often precedes complete obstruction. Partial airway obstruction can cause cerebral or pulmonary oedema, exhaustion, secondary apnoea, and hypoxic brain injury, and eventually cardiac arrest.

Central nervous system depression may cause loss of airway patency and protective reflexes. Causes include head injury and intracerebral disease, hypercarbia, the depressant effect of metabolic disorders (e.g. hypoglycaemia in diabetic patients), and drugs, including alcohol, opioids and general anaesthetic agents. Laryngospasm can occur with upper airway stimulation in a semi-conscious patient whose airway reflexes remain intact.

In some people, the upper airway can become obstructed when they sleep (obstructive sleep apnoea). This is more common in obese patients and obstruction can be made worse by other factors (e.g. sedative drugs).

Recognition of airway obstruction

Assess the patency of the airway in anyone at risk of obstruction. A conscious patient will complain of difficulty in breathing, may be choking, and will be distressed. With partial airway obstruction, efforts at breathing will be noisy. Complete airway obstruction is silent and there is no

Causes of airway obstruction

- Central nervous system depression
- Blood
- Vomitus
- Foreign body (e.g. tooth, food)
- Direct trauma to face or throat
- Epiglottitis
- Pharyngeal swelling (e.g. infection, oedema)
- Laryngospasm
- Bronchospasm – causes narrowing of the small airways in the lung
- Bronchial secretions
- Blocked tracheostomy or laryngectomy

air movement at the patient's mouth. Any respiratory movements are usually strenuous.

The accessory muscles of respiration will be involved, causing a 'see-saw' or 'rocking-horse' pattern of chest and abdominal movement: the chest is drawn in and the abdomen expands on inspiration, and the opposite occurs on expiration.

Treatment of airway obstruction

The priority is to ensure that the airway remains patent. Treat any problem that places the airway at risk; for example, suck blood and gastric contents from the airway and, unless contraindicated, turn the patient on their side. Give oxygen as soon as possible to achieve an arterial blood oxygen saturation by pulse oximetry (SpO_2) in the range of 94–98%.

Assume actual or impending airway obstruction in anyone with a depressed level of consciousness, regardless of cause. Take steps to safeguard the airway and prevent further complications such as aspiration of gastric contents. This may involve nursing the patient on their side or with a head-up tilt. Simple airway opening manoeuvres (head tilt/chin lift or jaw thrust), insertion of an oropharyngeal or nasal airway can improve airway patency. Tracheal intubation by an airway expert may be required. Consider insertion of a nasogastric tube to empty the stomach.

Breathing problems

Causes of breathing problems

Breathing inadequacy may be acute or chronic. It may be continuous or intermittent, and severe enough to cause the person to stop breathing (apnoea or respiratory arrest). This will rapidly lead to a secondary cardiac arrest if not treated.

Respiratory arrest often arises from a combination of factors. In a patient with chronic respiratory inadequacy, a chest infection, muscle weakness, or fractured ribs may lead to exhaustion, further depressing respiratory function. If breathing is insufficient to oxygenate the blood adequately, lack of oxygen to the vital organs will lead to loss of consciousness and eventually cardiac arrest.

Respiratory drive

Central nervous system depression can decrease or abolish respiratory drive. The causes are the same as those for airway obstruction from central nervous system depression.

Respiratory effort

The main respiratory muscles are the diaphragm and intercostal muscles. The latter are innervated at the level of their respective ribs and may be paralysed by a spinal cord lesion above this level. The innervation of the diaphragm is derived from the third, fourth and fifth segment of the spinal cord. Spontaneous breathing cannot occur with severe cervical cord damage above this level.

Inadequate respiratory effort, caused by muscle weakness or nerve damage, occurs with many diseases (e.g. myasthenia gravis, Guillain-Barré syndrome, and multiple sclerosis). Chronic malnourishment and severe long-term illness may also contribute to generalised weakness.

Breathing can also be impaired with restrictive chest wall abnormalities such as kyphoscoliosis. Pain from fractured ribs or sternum will prevent deep breaths and coughing.

Lung disorders

Severe lung disease will impair gas exchange. Causes include infection, exacerbation of chronic obstructive pulmonary disease (COPD), asthma, pulmonary embolus (PE), lung contusion, acute respiratory distress syndrome (ARDS) and pulmonary oedema. Lung function is also impaired by a pneumothorax or haemothorax. A tension pneumothorax impairs gas exchange and reduces venous return to the heart , and causes a decrease in blood pressure.

Recognition of breathing problems

A conscious patient will complain of shortness of breath and be distressed. The history and examination will usually indicate the underlying cause. Hypoxaemia and hypercarbia can cause irritability, confusion, lethargy and depressed consciousness. Cyanosis is a late sign. A fast respiratory rate (> 25 min^{-1}) is a useful, simple indicator of breathing problems. Pulse oximetry is an easy, non-invasive measure of the adequacy of oxygenation (Chapter 9). However, it is not a reliable indicator of ventilation and an arterial blood gas sample is necessary to obtain values for arterial carbon dioxide tension ($PaCO_2$) and pH. A rising $PaCO_2$ and a decrease in pH are often late signs in a patient with severe respiratory problems.

Treatment of breathing problems

Give oxygen to all acutely ill hypoxaemic patients and treat the underlying cause. Give oxygen at 15 L min^{-1} using a high-concentration reservoir mask. Once oxygen saturation can be measured reliably, change the oxygen mask and aim for a SpO_2 in the range of 94–98%. Give early IV antibiotics to a patient with a severe pneumonia or start bronchodilator (salbutamol nebulisers) and steroid treatment for a patient with severe asthma.

Patients who are having difficulty breathing or are becoming tired will need help with their breathing. Non-invasive ventilation using a face mask or high-flow nasal cannulae can be useful and prevent the need for tracheal intubation and ventilation. It is best to call for expert help early for patients who cannot breathe adequately as ICU admission for sedation, tracheal intubation and controlled ventilation may be needed.

Circulation problems

Causes of circulation problems

Circulation problems can be caused by primary heart disease or by heart abnormalities secondary to other problems. In acutely ill patients, circulation problems are most commonly caused by hypovolaemia. The heart may stop suddenly or may produce an inadequate cardiac output for a while before stopping.

Primary heart problems

Sudden cardiac arrest is most commonly caused by an arrhythmia secondary to an acute coronary syndrome – see below. The commonest initial cardiac arrest rhythm is ventricular fibrillation (VF).

Causes of ventricular fibrillation

- Acute coronary syndromes
- Hypertensive heart disease
- Valve disease
- Drugs (e.g. antiarrhythmic drugs, tricyclic antidepressants, digoxin)
- Inherited cardiac diseases (e.g. long QT syndromes)
- Acidosis
- Abnormal electrolyte concentration (e.g. potassium, magnesium, calcium)
- Hypothermia
- Electrocution

Acute coronary syndromes

Acute coronary syndromes (ACS) usually present with chest pain or discomfort resulting from myocardial ischaemia. The distinct categories are distinguished initially by the presence or absence of ST-segment elevation on a 12-lead ECG and, in those without ST-segment elevation, by the presence or absence of a raised blood troponin concentration suggesting myocardial injury:

- ST-segment-elevation myocardial infarction (STEMI)

- Non ST-segment-elevation acute coronary syndromes (NSTE ACS)

    - Non-ST- segment-elevation myocardial infarction (NSTEMI)

    - Unstable angina (UA).

Recognition of acute coronary syndromes

- Acute myocardial infarction (AMI) typically presents with chest pain that is felt as a heaviness or tightness or indigestion-like discomfort in the chest. The pain or discomfort often radiates into the neck or throat, into one or both arms (more commonly the left), and into the back or into the epigastrium. Some patients experience the discomfort more in one of these areas than in the chest.

- Sometimes discomfort is accompanied by belching, which can be misinterpreted as evidence of indigestion as the cause. A history of sustained (i.e. 20–30 minutes or more) acute chest pain typical of AMI, with acute ST-segment elevation on a 12-lead ECG is the basis for a diagnosis of STEMI.

- Some patients present with chest pain suggestive of AMI and less specific ECG abnormalities, such as ST segment depression or T wave inversion. A history suggestive of ACS and laboratory tests showing substantial release of troponin indicates that myocardial damage has occurred. This is referred to as NSTEMI.

- Consider unstable angina when there is an unprovoked and prolonged episode of chest pain, raising suspicion of AMI but without definite ECG or laboratory evidence of AMI.

- People with chest pain need urgent medical attention. Out of hospital they should dial 999 and call an ambulance. If they have an ACS they are at high risk of VF cardiac arrest and sudden cardiac death (SCD).

Initial treatment of acute coronary syndromes

Patients with an ACS should be closely monitored (e.g. on a coronary care unit). Immediate treatment for ACS comprises:

- aspirin 300 mg orally, crushed or chewed, as soon as possible

- sublingual glyceryl trinitrate (spray or tablet) unless the patient is hypotensive

- oxygen if the patient is hypoxic (saturation < 94% on air):

    - aim for saturation of 94–98%

    - in the presence of chronic obstructive pulmonary disease aim for 88–92%

- pain relief with IV opiate analgesia (morphine):

    - titrated to control symptoms whilst avoiding sedation and respiratory depression

    - given with an anti-emetic.

Refer urgently to a cardiologist for further treatment. Further common interventions include:

- Percutaneous coronary intervention (PCI) to re-open the occluded coronary artery. Primary PCI (PPCI) is the preferred treatment for STEMI.

- Antithrombotic agents (e.g. clopidogrel).

- Anticoagulation.

Sudden cardiac death out of hospital

Coronary artery disease is the commonest cause of SCD. Non-ischaemic cardiomyopathy and valvular disease account for some other SCD events. A small percentage of SCDs are caused by inherited abnormalities (e.g. long and short QT syndromes, Brugada syndrome, hypertrophic cardiomyopathy, arrhythmogenic right ventricular cardiomyopathy), and by congenital heart disease.

In patients with a known diagnosis of cardiac disease, syncope (with or without a prodrome – particularly recent or recurrent) is as an independent risk factor for increased risk of death. Apparently healthy children and young adults who have SCD can also have symptoms and signs (e.g. syncope/pre-syncope, chest pain, palpitation, heart murmur) that should alert healthcare professionals to seek expert help to prevent cardiac arrest.

Features that indicate a high probability of arrhythmic syncope include:

- syncope in the supine position (i.e. fainting when already lying down)

- syncope occurring during or after exercise (although syncope after exercise is often vasovagal)

- syncope with no or only brief prodromal symptoms (e.g. sudden collapse without warning signs)

- repeated episodes of unexplained syncope

- syncope in individuals with a family history of sudden death or inherited cardiac condition.

Assessment in a clinic specialising in the care of those at risk for SCD is recommended in family members of young victims of SCD or those with a known cardiac disorder resulting in an increased risk of SCD. Specific and detailed guidance for the care of individuals with transient loss of consciousness is available (http://guidance.nice.org.uk/CG109).

Secondary heart problems
The heart is affected by changes elsewhere in the body. For example, cardiac arrest will occur rapidly following asphyxia from airway obstruction or apnoea, or after acute severe blood loss. Severe hypoxia and anaemia, hypothermia, oligaemia and severe septic shock will also impair cardiac function and this can lead to cardiac arrest.

Recognition of secondary heart problems
The signs and symptoms of cardiac disease include chest pain, shortness of breath, syncope, tachycardia, bradycardia, tachypnoea (high respiratory rate), hypotension, poor peripheral perfusion (prolonged capillary refill time), altered mental state, and oliguria (low urine output).

Most SCDs occur in people with pre-existing cardiac disease, which may have been unrecognised. Asymptomatic or silent cardiac disease includes hypertensive heart disease, aortic valve disease, cardiomyopathy, myocarditis, and coronary disease.

Treatment of secondary heart problems
Treat the underlying cause of circulatory failure. In many sick patients, this means giving oxygen to correct hypoxaemia and intravenous fluids to correct hypovolaemia.

The ABCDE approach

Underlying principles
The approach to all deteriorating or critically ill patients is the same. The underlying principles are:

1. Use the **A**irway, **B**reathing, **C**irculation, **D**isability, **E**xposure approach to assess and treat the patient.

2. Do a complete initial assessment and re-assess regularly.

3. Treat life-threatening problems before moving to the next part of assessment.

4. Assess the effects of treatment.

5. Recognise when you need extra help. Call for help early.

6. Use all team members. This enables several interventions (e.g. assessment, attaching monitors, intravenous access) to be undertaken simultaneously.

7. Communicate effectively – use SBAR or RSVP (Chapter 1).

8. The aim is to keep the patient alive, and achieve some clinical improvement. This will buy time for further treatment and making a diagnosis.

9. Keep calm. Remember – it can take a few minutes for treatments to work.

10. Use the ABCDE approach irrespective of your training and experience in clinical assessment and treatment. The detail of your assessment and which treatments you give will depend on your role, clinical knowledge and skills. If you recognise a problem or are unsure make sure you have called for help early.

First steps

1. Ensure personal safety. Wear apron and gloves as appropriate.

2. Your first impression is important. Look at the patient in general to see if the patient 'looks unwell'.

3. If he is awake, ask "How are you?" and hold his hand. If he appears unconscious or has collapsed, shake him and ask "Are you alright?" If he responds by talking normally he has a patent airway, is breathing and has brain perfusion. If he speaks only in short sentences, he may have breathing problems. If he does not respond this is concerning as he is likely to be critically ill.

4. This first rapid 'Look, Listen and Feel" of the patient should take about 30 seconds and will often tell you a patient is critically ill and there is a need for urgent help. Ask a colleague to ensure appropriate help is coming.

5. Monitor the vital signs early. Attach a pulse oximeter, ECG monitor and a non-invasive blood pressure monitor to all critically ill patients, as soon as possible.

6. Insert an intravenous cannula as soon as possible. Take bloods for investigation when inserting the intravenous cannula.

7. If the patient is unconscious, unresponsive, and is not breathing normally (occasional gasps are not normal and are a sign of cardiac arrest) start CPR according to the guidance in Chapter 3. If you have any doubts about the diagnosis of cardiac arrest, start CPR whilst waiting for expert help to arrive.

Airway (A)

Airway obstruction is an emergency. Get expert help immediately.

1. Look for the signs of airway obstruction:

   • Airway obstruction causes paradoxical chest and abdominal movements ('see-saw' respirations) and the use of the accessory muscles of respiration. Central cyanosis (e.g. blue lips and tongue) is a late sign of airway obstruction. In complete airway obstruction, there are no breath sounds at the mouth or nose. In partial obstruction, air entry is diminished and often noisy.

   • In the critically ill patient, depressed consciousness often leads to airway obstruction, especially if he is laying flat on his back, or he is sitting-up and his head has fallen forwards.

2. Airway obstruction is a medical emergency and requires immediate treatment:

   • In most cases, simple methods of airway clearance are all that are required (e.g. airway opening manoeuvres, suction of the airway, insertion of an oropharyngeal or nasopharyngeal airway). Advanced airway techniques such as tracheal intubation by an expert can be required when these fail.

3. Give oxygen at high concentration:

   • Give high-concentration oxygen using a mask with oxygen reservoir. Ensure that the oxygen flow is sufficient (usually 15 L min^{-1}) to prevent collapse of the reservoir during inspiration.

   • Adjust the amount of oxygen given by monitoring the oxygen saturation with a pulse oximeter. Aim to maintain an oxygen saturation of 94–98%. In patients at risk of hypercapnic respiratory failure (see below) aim for an oxygen saturation of 88–92%.

Breathing (B)

Diagnose and treat immediately life-threatening conditions early (e.g. acute severe asthma, pulmonary oedema, tension pneumothorax, and massive haemothorax).

1. Look, listen and feel for the general signs of respiratory distress: sweating, central cyanosis, use of the accessory muscles of respiration, and abdominal breathing.

2. Count the respiratory rate. The normal rate is 12–20 breaths min^{-1}. A high (> 25 min^{-1}) or increasing respiratory rate is a marker of illness and a warning that the patient may deteriorate suddenly.

3. Assess the depth of each breath, the pattern (rhythm) of respiration and whether chest expansion is equal and normal on both sides.

4. Note any chest deformity (this can increase the risk of deterioration in the ability to breathe normally). Note the presence and patency of any chest drains. Remember that abdominal distension can limit diaphragmatic movement, thereby worsening respiratory distress.

5. Record the inspired oxygen concentration (%) and the SpO$_2$ reading of the pulse oximeter. The pulse oximeter measures blood oxygen saturation only. If the patient is receiving supplemental oxygen, the SpO$_2$ may be normal even with inadequate ventilation and hypercapnia (a raised level of carbon dioxide in the blood and an indicator of respiratory failure).

6. Listen to the patient's breath sounds a short distance from his face: rattling airway noises indicate the presence of airway secretions, usually because the patient cannot cough or take a deep breath. Audible stridor (an upper airway noise on breathing in) or wheeze (on expiration) suggests partial, but significant, airway obstruction.

7. Percuss the chest if you are trained to do so: hyper-resonance suggests a pneumothorax; dullness usually indicates consolidation or pleural fluid.

8. Auscultate the chest with a stethoscope if you are trained to do so: bronchial breathing indicates lung consolidation with patent airways; absent or reduced sounds suggest a pneumothorax or pleural fluid or lung consolidation caused by complete obstruction.

9. Check the position of the trachea in the suprasternal notch: deviation to one side indicates mediastinal shift (e.g. pneumothorax, lung fibrosis or pleural fluid). Tracheal deviation is often difficult to identify even for experts.

10. Feel the chest wall to detect surgical emphysema or crepitus (suggesting a pneumothorax until proven otherwise).

11. The treatment of respiratory disorders depends upon the cause. All critically ill patients should be given oxygen. In some patients with chronic obstructive pulmonary disease (COPD), high concentrations of oxygen can depress breathing (i.e. they are at risk of hypercapnic respiratory failure – often referred to as type 2 respiratory failure). Nevertheless, these patients will also sustain end-organ damage or cardiac arrest if their blood oxygen level is allowed to decrease. In this group, aim for a lower than normal oxygen saturation. Give oxygen via a Venturi 28% mask (4 L min^{-1}) or a

24% Venturi mask (4 L min⁻¹) initially and reassess. Aim for target SpO₂ range of 88–92% in most COPD patients, but evaluate the target for each patient based on the patient's arterial blood gas measurements during previous exacerbations (if available). Some patients with chronic lung disease carry an oxygen alert card (that documents their target saturation) and their own appropriate Venturi mask.

12. If the patient's depth or rate of breathing is inadequate, or absent, use two-person bag-mask, or pocket mask ventilation to improve oxygenation and ventilation, whilst calling immediately for expert help. In cooperative patients who do not have airway obstruction consider the use of non-invasive ventilation (NIV). In patients with an acute exacerbation of COPD, the use of NIV is often helpful and prevents the need for tracheal intubation and invasive ventilation.

Circulation (C)

In almost all medical and surgical emergencies, consider hypovolaemia to be the likeliest cause of shock, unless proven otherwise. Unless there are obvious signs of a cardiac cause (e.g. chest pain, heart failure), give intravenous fluid to any patient with cool peripheries and a fast heart rate.

In surgical patients, rapidly exclude bleeding (overt or hidden). Remember that breathing problems, such as a tension pneumothorax, can also compromise a patient's circulatory state. This should have been treated earlier on in the assessment.

1. Look at the colour of the hands and fingers: are they blue, pink, pale or mottled?

2. Hold the patient's hand: is it cool or warm?

3. Measure the capillary refill time (CRT). Apply pressure for 5 seconds on a fingertip held at heart level (or just above) with enough pressure to cause blanching. Time how long it takes for the skin to return to the colour of the surrounding skin after releasing the pressure. The normal value for CRT is usually less than 2 seconds. A prolonged CRT suggests poor peripheral perfusion. Other factors (e.g. cold surroundings, poor lighting, old age) can prolong CRT.

4. Count the patient's pulse rate (or preferably heart rate by listening to the heart with a stethoscope).

5. Feel the peripheral and central (carotid) pulses, assessing for presence, rate, quality, regularity and equality. Barely palpable central pulses suggest a poor cardiac output, whilst a bounding pulse can indicate sepsis.

6. Measure the patient's blood pressure. Even in shock, the blood pressure may be normal, because compensatory mechanisms increase peripheral resistance in response to reduced cardiac output. A low diastolic blood pressure suggests arterial vasodilation

(as in anaphylaxis or sepsis). A narrowed pulse pressure (difference between systolic and diastolic pressures; normally 35–45 mmHg) suggests arterial vasoconstriction (cardiogenic shock or hypovolaemia).

7. Auscultate the heart with a stethoscope if you are trained to do so. Is there a murmur or pericardial rub? Are the heart sounds difficult to hear? Does the audible heart rate correspond to the pulse rate?

8. Look for other signs of a poor cardiac output, such as reduced conscious level and, if the patient has a urinary catheter, oliguria (urine volume less than 0.5 mL kg⁻¹ h⁻¹).

9. Look thoroughly for external bleeding from wounds or drains or evidence of concealed bleeding (e.g. thoracic, intra-peritoneal, retroperitoneal or into gut). Intra-thoracic, intra-abdominal or pelvic blood loss can be significant, even if drains are empty.

10. The treatment of cardiovascular collapse depends on the cause, but should be directed at fluid replacement, bleeding control and restoration of tissue perfusion. Seek the signs of conditions that are immediately life threatening (e.g. cardiac tamponade, massive or continuing bleeding, septicaemic shock) and treat them urgently.

11. Insert one or more large (14 or 16 G) intravenous cannulae. Use short, wide-bore cannulae, because they enable the highest flow.

12. Take blood from the cannula for routine haematological, biochemical, coagulation and microbiological investigations, and cross-matching, before infusing intravenous fluid.

13. Give a rapid bolus of 500 mL of warmed crystalloid solution (e.g. Hartmann's solution or 0.9% sodium chloride) over less than 15 minutes. Use smaller volumes (e.g. 250 mL) for patients with known cardiac failure or trauma and use closer monitoring (listen to the chest for crackles after each bolus).

14. Reassess the heart rate and BP regularly (every 5 minutes), aiming for the patient's normal BP or, if this is unknown, a target > 100 mmHg systolic.

15. If the patient does not improve, repeat the fluid challenge. Seek expert help if there is a lack of response to repeated fluid boluses. Lack of response can indicate bleeding.

16. If symptoms and signs of cardiac failure (dyspnoea, increased heart rate, raised JVP, a third heart sound and pulmonary crackles on auscultation) occur, decrease the fluid infusion rate or stop the fluids altogether. Ask for expert help as other treatments that improve tissue perfusion (e.g. inotropes or vasopressors) may be needed.

17. If the patient has chest pain and a suspected ACS, record a 12-lead ECG early, and treat initially with aspirin, nitroglycerine, oxygen, and morphine.

18. Immediate general treatment for ACS includes:

- aspirin 300 mg orally, crushed or chewed, as soon as possible; sublingual glyceryl trinitrate (spray or tablet) unless the patient is hypotensive;

- oxygen if the patient is hypoxic (saturation < 94% on air):

  - aim for saturation of 94–98%

  - in the presence of COPD aim for 88–92%

- pain relief with IV opiate analgesia (morphine):

  - titrated to control symptoms whilst avoiding sedation and respiratory depression

  - given with an anti-emetic.

Disability (D)

Common causes of unconsciousness include profound hypoxia, hypercapnia, cerebral hypoperfusion due to a low blood pressure, or sedatives or analgesic drugs.

1. Review and treat the ABCs: exclude or treat hypoxia and hypotension.

2. Check the patient's drug chart for reversible drug-induced causes of depressed consciousness. Give an antagonist where appropriate (e.g. naloxone for opioid toxicity).

3. Examine the pupils (size, equality and reaction to light).

4. Make a rapid initial assessment of the patient's conscious level using the AVPU method: **A**lert, responds to **V**ocal stimuli, responds to **P**ainful stimuli or **U**nresponsive to all stimuli. Alternatively, use the Glasgow Coma Scale score. A painful stimuli can be given by squeezing the trapezius muscle, or by applying supra-orbital pressure (at the supraorbital notch) or pressure on a finger nail.

5. Measure the blood glucose to exclude hypoglycaemia using a rapid finger-prick bedside testing method. In the sickest patients blood should be taken from a vein or artery as finger prick samples may not be reliable for blood glucose measurements. Follow local protocols for management of hypoglycaemia. For example, if the blood sugar is below 4.0 mmol L^{-1} in an unconscious patient, give an initial dose of 50 mL of 10% glucose solution intravenously. If necessary, give further doses of intravenous 10% glucose every minute until the patient has fully regained consciousness, or a total of 250 mL of 10% glucose has been given. Repeat blood glucose measurements to monitor the effects of treatment. If there is no improvement consider further doses of 10% glucose. Specific national guidance exists for the management of hypoglycaemia in adults with diabetes mellitus.

6. Nurse unconscious patients in the lateral position if their airway is not protected.

Exposure (E)

To examine the patient properly full exposure of the body may be necessary. Respect the patient's dignity and minimise heat loss.

Additional information

1. Take a full clinical history from the patient, any relatives or friends, and other staff.

2. Review the patient's notes and charts:

   - Study both absolute and trended values of vital signs.

   - Check that important routine medications are prescribed and being given.

3. Review the results of laboratory or radiological investigations.

4. Consider which level of care is required by the patient (e.g. ward, HDU, ICU).

5. Make complete entries in the patient's notes of your findings, assessment and treatment. Where necessary, handover the patient to your colleagues using SBAR or RSVP.

6. Record the patient's response to therapy.

7. Consider definitive treatment of the patient's underlying condition.

8. Keep the patient and relatives informed of what is happening.

Summary learning

- **Most patients who have an in-hospital cardiac arrest have warning signs and symptoms before the arrest.**

- **Early recognition and treatment of the deteriorating patient will prevent some cardiorespiratory arrests.**

- **Use strategies such as early warning scoring (EWS) systems to identify patients at risk of cardiorespiratory arrest.**

- **Airway, breathing and circulation problems can cause cardiorespiratory arrest.**

- **Use the ABCDE approach to assess and treat critically ill patients.**

My key take-home messages from this chapter

Further reading

National Early Warning Score (NEWS) 2: Standardising the assessment of acute-illness severity in the NHS. Updated report of a working party. Royal College of Physicians, London, 2017.

NICE clinical guideline 50 Acutely ill patients in hospital: recognition of and response to acute illness in adults in hospital. London: National Institute for Health and Clinical Excellence; 2007.
https://www.nice.org.uk/guidance/cg50

National Institute for Health and Care Excellence. Clinical Guideline 167. Myocardial infarction with ST-segment elevation: The acute management of myocardial infarction with ST-segment elevation. NICE 2013.
www.nice.org.uk/Guidance

National Institute for Health and Care Excellence. Clinical Guideline 94. Unstable angina and NSTEMI: The early management of unstable angina and non-ST-segment-elevation myocardial infarction. NICE 2010.
www.nice.org.uk/Guidance

National Institute for Health and Care Excellence. Clinical Guideline 172. Myocardial infarction: secondary prevention. Secondary prevention in primary and secondary care for patients following a myocardial infarction. NICE 2013. www.nice.org.uk/Guidance

Smith GB. In-hospital cardiac arrest: Is it time for an in-hospital 'chain of prevention'? Resuscitation 2010:81:1209-11.

Soar J, Callaway CW, Aibiki M, et al. Part 4: Advanced life support: 2015 International Consensus on Cardiopulmonary Resuscitation and Emergency Cardiovascular Care Science With Treatment Recommendations. Resuscitation 2015;95:e71-e122.

Soar J, Nolan JP, Bottiger BW, et al. European Resuscitation Council Guidelines for Resuscitation 2015 Section 3 Adult Advanced Life Support. Resuscitation 2015;95:99-146.

The Hospital Management of Hypoglycaemia in Adults with Diabetes Mellitus. Joint British Diabetes Societies. Revised 2013.

In-hospital resuscitation

Contents

- **Features specific to in-hospital resuscitation**
- **Sequence for the collapsed patient in hospital**

Learning outcomes

To enable you to:

- **Start resuscitation in hospital**
- **Give high quality cardiopulmonary resuscitation (CPR) with minimal interruption**
- **Continue resuscitation until more experienced help arrives**

Introduction

After in-hospital cardiac arrest, the division between basic life support and advanced life support is arbitrary. The public expect that all clinical staff know how to do cardiopulmonary resuscitation (CPR). For every in-hospital cardiac arrests, ensure that:

- cardiorespiratory arrest is recognised immediately

- help is summoned using a standard telephone number (2222 in the UK)

- CPR is started immediately and, if indicated, defibrillation is attempted as soon as possible (within 3 minutes).

This chapter is primarily for healthcare professionals who are first to respond to an in-hospital cardiac arrest, but is also applicable to healthcare professionals working in other clinical settings.

Why is in-hospital resuscitation different?

The exact sequence of actions after in-hospital cardiac arrest depends on:

- location (clinical/non clinical area; monitored/unmonitored area)

- skills of the first responders

- number of responders

- equipment available

- hospital response system to cardiac arrest and medical emergencies (e.g. medical emergency team (MET), resuscitation team).

Location of cardiac arrest

Patients who have a witnessed or monitored cardiac arrest in a critical care area are usually diagnosed and treated quickly. Ideally, all patients who are at high risk of cardiac arrest should be cared for in a monitored area where staff and facilities for immediate resuscitation are available. Patients, visitors or staff may also have a cardiac arrest in

ILS

non-clinical areas (e.g. car parks, corridors). You may have to move the patient to enable effective resuscitation. Guidance from the Resuscitation Council (UK) for safer handling during resuscitation in healthcare settings is available:

https://www.resus.org.uk/publications/guidance-for-safer-handling-during-cpr-in-healthcare-settings/.

Skills of first responders

All staff should be able to recognise cardiac arrest, call for help and start resuscitation. They should do what they have been trained to do. For example, if you work in critical care and emergency medicine you may have more advanced resuscitation skills and greater experience in resuscitation than those who use resuscitation skills rarely. Hospital staff who respond to a cardiac arrest may have different levels of skill to manage the airway, breathing and circulation. Use the skills you are trained to do.

Number of responders

If you are alone, always make sure that help is coming. Usually, staff colleagues are nearby and several actions can be undertaken simultaneously. Hospital staffing tends to be at its lowest during the night and at weekends. This can influence patient monitoring, treatment and outcomes. Studies show that survival rates from in-hospital cardiac arrest are lower during nights and weekends.

Equipment available

Staff should have immediate access to resuscitation equipment and drugs. Ideally, the equipment used for cardiopulmonary resuscitation (including defibrillators) and the layout of equipment and drugs should be the same throughout the hospital. You should be familiar with the resuscitation equipment used in your clinical area.

Serious patient safety incidents associated with CPR and patient deterioration are commonly associated with equipment problems during resuscitation (e.g. portable suction not working, defibrillator pads missing). Specially designed trolleys or sealed tray systems can improve speed of access to equipment and reduce adverse incidents. Resuscitation equipment checked on a regular basis to ensure it is ready for use.

Defibrillators with automated rhythm recognition (automated external defibrillator (AED)) can be used in clinical and non-clinical areas where staff do not have rhythm recognition skills, or rarely need to use a defibrillator. Manual defibrillation used by trained staff is associated with increased survival after in-hospital cardiac arrest. Use an AED when someone trained to use a manual defibrillator is not immediately available, or when only an AED is available.

Waveform capnography is a monitor that is always used during anaesthesia and for critically ill patients requiring mechanical ventilation. It must be used to confirm correct tracheal tube placement during resuscitation and can also help guide resuscitation interventions (Chapter 4).

Waveform capnography monitoring is available on newer defibrillators, as part of portable monitors or as a hand-held device.

After successful resuscitation, patients often need transferring to other clinical areas (e.g. intensive care unit) or other hospitals. Ensure transfer equipment and drugs are available to enable this.

At the end of every resuscitation attempt, ensure equipment and drugs are replaced and available to use next time they are needed.

Resuscitation team

The resuscitation team can be a traditional cardiac arrest team, which is called only when cardiac arrest is recognised. In some hospitals a resuscitation team (e.g. medical emergency team (MET)) is called if a patient is deteriorating before cardiac arrest occurs.

Resuscitation team members should meet for introductions and plan before they attend actual events. Knowing each other's names, backgrounds and discussing how the team will work together during a resuscitation will improve team work during resuscitation attempts. Team members should debrief after each event, to enable performance and concerns to be discussed openly. This has most benefit when discussions are based on data collected during the event.

Sequence for collapsed patient in a hospital

An algorithm for the initial management of in-hospital cardiac arrest is shown in Figure 3.1.

1 Ensure personal safety

- There are very few reports of harm to rescuers during resuscitation.

- Your own safety and that of resuscitation team members is the first priority.

- Check that the patient's surroundings are safe.

- Put on gloves as soon as possible. Other personal protective equipment (PPE) (e.g. eye protection, face masks, aprons, gowns) may be necessary especially when the patient has a serious infection such as tuberculosis. Follow local infection control measures to minimise risks.

- The actual risk of infection to rescuers during CPR is much lower than perceived. There are very rare reports of infections such as tuberculosis (TB), and severe acute respiratory distress syndrome (SARS). Transmission of HIV during CPR has never been reported.

- Be careful with sharps; a sharps box must be available.

- Use safe handling techniques for moving victims during resuscitation.

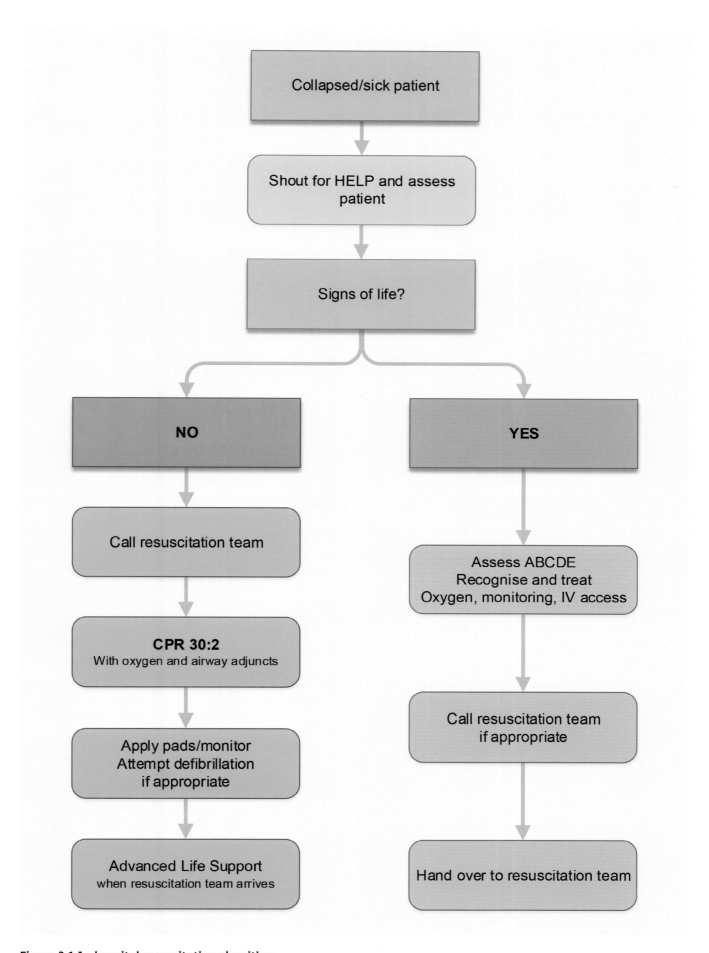

Figure 3.1 In-hospital resuscitation algorithm

- Avoid contact with corrosive chemicals (e.g. strong acids, alkalis, paraquat) or substances such as organophosphates that are easily absorbed through the skin or respiratory tract.

2 Check the patient for a response

- If you see a patient collapse or find a patient apparently unconscious first shout for help, then assess if he is responsive (shake and shout). Gently shake his shoulders and ask loudly: "Are you all right?" (Figure 3.2).

- If other members of staff are nearby it will be possible to undertake actions simultaneously.

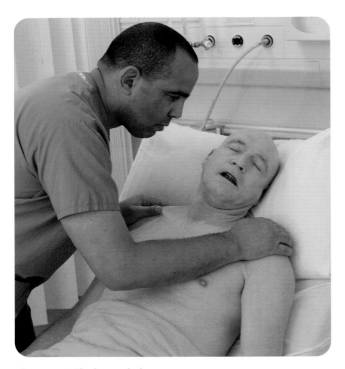

Figure 3.2 Shake and shout

3A If he responds

- Urgent medical assessment is required. Call for help according to local protocols. This may include calling a resuscitation team (e.g. MET).

- While waiting for the team, assess the patient using the ABCDE (Airway, Breathing, Circulation, Disability, Exposure) approach (Chapter 2).

- Give oxygen. Use a pulse oximeter to help adjust how much oxygen you give (Chapter 9).

- Attach monitoring: a minimum of pulse oximetry, ECG and blood pressure. Record the vital signs and calculate the early warning score (EWS).

- Obtain venous access, and take blood samples for investigation.

- Prepare for handover using SBAR (Situation, Background, Assessment, Recommendation) or RSVP (Reason, Story, Vital signs, Plan).

3B If he does not respond

The exact sequence will depend on your training and experience in assessment of breathing and circulation in sick patients.

- Shout for help (if not done already).

- Turn the patient on to his back.

- Take 10 seconds at most to determine if the patient is in cardiac arrest.

- Open the airway using head tilt and chin lift (Figure 3.3).

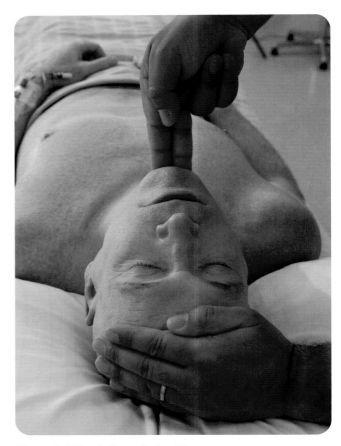

Figure 3.3 Head tilt and chin lift

- If there is a risk of cervical spine injury, use a jaw thrust or chin lift in combination with manual in-line stabilisation of the head and neck by an assistant (if enough people are available). If life-threatening airway obstruction persists despite effective application of jaw thrust or chin lift, add head tilt a small amount at a time until the airway is open; establishing a patent airway, oxygenation and ventilation must take priority over concerns about a cervical spine injury.

- Keeping the airway open, LOOK, LISTEN, and FEEL (Figure 3.4) to determine if the victim is breathing normally. This is a rapid check and should **take less than 10 seconds:**

  - Look for chest movement (breathing or coughing).

  - Look for any other movement or signs of life.

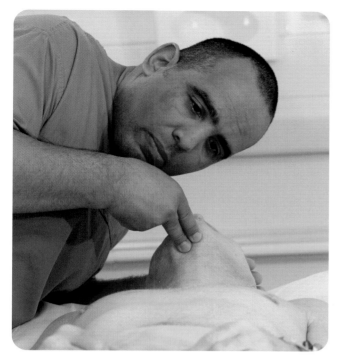

Figure 3.4 Assessing for breathing and signs of life

- Listen at the victim's mouth for breath sounds.

- Feel for air on your cheek.

• If trained and experienced in the assessment of sick patients, check for breathing and assess the carotid pulse at the same time (Figure 3.5).

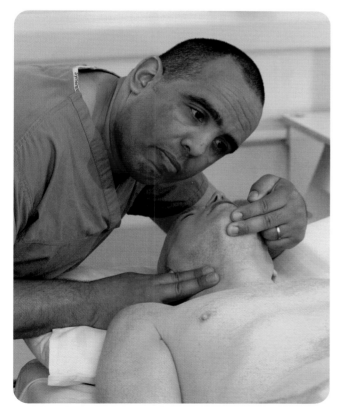

Figure 3.5 Simultaneous check for breathing, pulse and signs of life

• Agonal breathing (occasional, irregular gasps) is common in the early stages of cardiac arrest and is a sign of cardiac arrest and should not be confused as a sign of life/circulation. Agonal breathing and limb movement can also occur during chest compressions as cerebral perfusion improves, but is not indicative of a return of spontaneous circulation (ROSC).

• If the patient has no signs of life (based on lack of purposeful movement, normal breathing, coughing), or there is any doubt, start CPR (step 4B below) until more help arrives or the patient shows signs of life.

• Diagnosing cardiac arrest can be difficult. If unsure, do not delay starting CPR. The patient is far more likely to die if there is a delay diagnosing cardiac arrest and starting CPR. Starting CPR on a very sick patient with a low blood pressure is unlikely to be harmful and may help.

• Assess the patient to confirm cardiac arrest even if the patient is monitored in a critical care area.

4A If he has a pulse or other signs of life

• Urgent medical assessment is required. Depending on the local protocols, this may take the form of a resuscitation team. While awaiting the team, assess and treat the patient using the ABCDE approach, give oxygen, attach monitoring and insert an intravenous cannula.

• Follow the steps in 3A above whilst waiting for the team.

• The patient is at high risk of further deterioration and cardiac arrest and needs continued observation until the team arrives.

4B If he has no pulse or signs of life

• Start CPR.

• Get a colleague to call the resuscitation team (Figure 3.6) and collect the resuscitation equipment and a defibrillator.

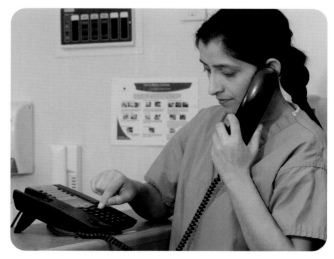

Figure 3.6 Call 2222 for the resuscitation team

- If alone, leave the patient to get help and equipment.

- Give 30 chest compressions followed by 2 ventilations.

- The correct hand position for chest compression is the middle of the lower half of the sternum.

- This hand position can be found quickly if you have been taught to 'place the heel of one hand in the centre of the chest with the other hand on top' and your teaching included a demonstration of placing hands in the middle of the lower half of the sternum (Figure 3.7).

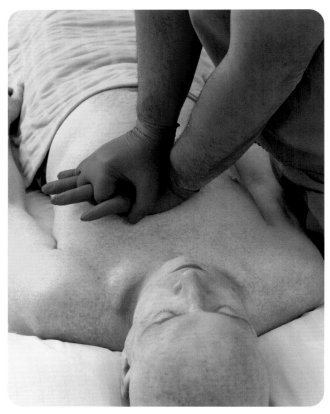

Figure 3.7 Hand position for chest compressions – place hands in the centre of the chest (middle of the lower half of the sternum)

- Ensure high quality chest compressions:

  - Depth of 5–6 cm

  - Rate of 100–120 compressions per minute

  - Allow the chest to recoil completely after each compression

  - Take approximately the same amount for time for compression and relaxation

  - Minimise any interruptions to chest compression (hands-off time).

- If available, use a prompt and/or feedback device to help ensure high quality chest compressions. Do not feel for pulses to assess the effectiveness of chest compressions.

- Each time compressions are resumed, place your hands without delay in the centre of the chest.

- The person doing chest compressions will get tired. If there are enough rescuers, this person should change about every 2 minutes or earlier if unable to maintain high quality chest compressions. Ensure this change is done with minimal interruption to compressions. This should be done during planned pauses in chest compression such as during rhythm assessment.

- Use whatever equipment is available immediately for airway and ventilation; for example, a pocket mask with an oral airway and oxygen, or two-person self-inflating bag-mask (Figure 3.8), or a supraglottic airway (e.g. laryngeal mask airway (LMA) or i-gel) and bag. In practice patients can have several airway techniques used stepwise during a cardiac arrest as equipment arrives and according to the skills of the rescuer.

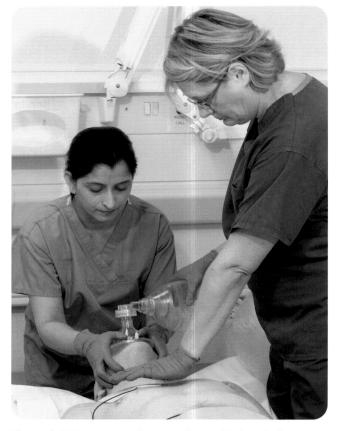

Figure 3.8 Two-person bag-mask ventilation during 30:2 CPR

- If airway and ventilation equipment are unavailable, consider mouth-to-mouth ventilation. If there are clinical reasons to avoid mouth-to-mouth contact, or you are unable to do this, do chest compressions until help or airway equipment arrives. There are usually good clinical reasons to avoid mouth-to-mouth ventilation in clinical settings, and it is therefore rarely used, but there will be situations where giving mouth-to-mouth breaths could be life saving. A pocket mask or bag-mask should be immediately available in all clinical areas. A pocket mask with filter, or a barrier device with one-way valve will minimise infection risk during rescue breathing.

- Irrespective of how you ventilate the patient's lungs, use an inspiratory time of about 1 second and give enough volume to produce a visible rise of the chest wall. Add supplemental oxygen as soon as possible.

- Avoid rapid or forceful breaths.

- Tracheal intubation should be attempted only by those who are trained, competent and experienced in this skill, and can insert the tracheal tube with minimal interruption (less than 5 seconds) to chest compressions.

- Waveform capnography must be used routinely for confirming that a tracheal tube is in the patient's airway and for subsequent monitoring during CPR. Once the patient's trachea has been intubated, continue chest compressions uninterrupted (except for defibrillation or pulse checks when indicated), at a rate of 100–120 min^{-1}, and ventilate the lungs at approximately 10 breaths min^{-1} (i.e. do not stop chest compressions for ventilation). If a supraglottic airway (e.g. LMA or i-gel) device has been inserted it may also be possible to ventilate the patient's lungs without stopping chest compressions.

- When the defibrillator arrives, apply self-adhesive defibrillation electrodes (pads) to the patient and analyse the rhythm. Apply the pads whilst chest compressions are ongoing (Figure 3.9). Self-adhesive electrode pads will enable faster assessment of heart rhythm than attaching ECG electrodes.

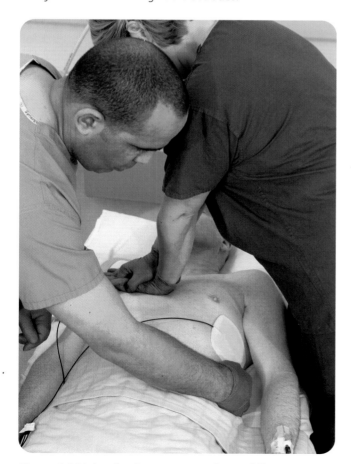

Figure 3.9 Maintain chest compressions whilst defibrillator pads are applied

- You may have an automated external defibrillator (AED), a manual defibrillator, or a defibrillator that has both an AED and manual mode.

- If you are not skilled in rhythm recognition use an AED (or AED mode). Switch on the AED and follow the audio-visual prompts.

- If you are experienced and confident in rhythm recognition use a manual defibrillator (or manual mode).

- If using a manual defibrillator, further treatments will depend on the cardiac arrest rhythm. See Chapter 4 for treatment of the different cardiac arrest rhythms.

- Continue resuscitation until the resuscitation team arrives or the patient shows signs of life.

- Once resuscitation is underway, and if there are sufficient staff present, prepare intravenous cannulae and drugs likely to be used by the resuscitation team (e.g. adrenaline).

- Use a clock for timing between rhythm checks. It is difficult to keep track of the number of 30:2 cycles. In practice, rhythm checks should take place about every 2 minutes and exact timing is not essential.

- The importance of uninterrupted chest compressions cannot be over emphasised. Even short interruptions to chest compressions may impact outcome. Make every effort to ensure that continuous, effective chest compressions are maintained throughout the resuscitation attempt.

- Plan exactly what you are going to do before stopping compressions to minimise the duration of the pause in compressions. Identify one person to be responsible for handover to the resuscitation team leader. Use SBAR or RSVP for handover (Chapter 1). Locate the patient's records.

4C If he is not breathing and has a pulse (respiratory arrest)

- Ventilate the patient's lungs (as described above) and check for a pulse every 10 breaths (about every minute).

- This diagnosis can be made only if you are confident in assessing breathing and pulse, and the patient has other signs of life (e.g. warm and well perfused, normal capillary refill).

- If there are any doubts about the presence of a pulse, start chest compressions until more experienced help arrives.

- All patients in respiratory arrest will develop cardiac arrest if the respiratory arrest is not treated rapidly and effectively.

5 If the patient has a monitored and witnessed cardiac arrest

If a patient has a monitored and witnessed cardiac arrest in the catheter laboratory, coronary care unit, a critical care area, or whilst monitored after cardiac surgery, and a manual defibrillator is rapidly available, or the patient is already connected to the defibrillator:

- Confirm cardiac arrest and shout for help.

- If the initial rhythm is ventricular fibrillation/pulseless ventricular tachycardia (VF/pVT), give up to three quick successive (stacked) shocks

- Rapidly check for a rhythm change and, if appropriate check for a pulse and other signs of ROSC after each defibrillation attempt.

- Start CPR if the third shock is unsuccessful.

You can do this only if you know how to use a manual defibrillator.

Summary learning

- **The exact sequence of actions after in-hospital cardiac arrest depends on the location, skills of the first responders, number of responders, equipment available, and the hospital response system to cardiac arrest and medical emergencies.**

- **Check for responsiveness, normal breathing, and signs of life to confirm cardiac arrest. This should take less than 10 seconds. Call for help and start CPR with chest compressions.**

- **Deliver high quality chest compressions with a depth of 5–6 cm, rate of 100–120 min^{-1}.**

- **Minimise interruptions to chest compressions for other interventions – this means all interruptions must be planned before stopping compressions.**

My key take-home messages from this chapter

Further reading

Nolan JP, Soar J, Smith GB, et al. Incidence and outcome of in-hospital cardiac arrest in the United Kingdom National Cardiac Arrest Audit. Resuscitation 2014;85:987-92.

Perkins GD, Handley AJ, Koster RM et al. Part 2: Adult basic life support and automated external defibrillation. Resuscitation 2015;95:81-98.

Resuscitation Council (UK). Guidance for safer handling during resuscitation in healthcare settings. July 2015.
https://www.resus.org.uk/publications/guidance-for-safer-handling-during-cpr-in-healthcare-settings/

Resuscitation Council (UK). Quality standards for cardiopulmonary resuscitation and training. https://www.resus.org.uk/quality-standards/

Soar J, Callaway CW, Aibiki M, et al. Part 4: Advanced life support: 2015 International Consensus on Cardiopulmonary Resuscitation and Emergency Cardiovascular Care Science With Treatment Recommendations. Resuscitation 2015;95:e71-e122.

Soar J, Nolan JP, Bottiger BW, et al. European Resuscitation Council Guidelines for Resuscitation 2015 Section 3 Adult Advanced Life Support. Resuscitation 2015;95:99-146.

Advanced Life Support algorithm

Contents

- **The Advanced Life Support (ALS) algorithm**
- **Shockable and non-shockable rhythms**

Learning outcomes

To enable you to:

- **Follow the ALS algorithm**
- **Understand the importance of minimally interrupted high quality chest compressions**
- **Treat shockable and non-shockable rhythms**
- **Consider potentially reversible causes of cardiac arrest**

Introduction

Heart rhythms associated with cardiac arrest are divided into two groups:

- shockable rhythms (ventricular fibrillation/pulseless ventricular tachycardia (VF/pVT)

- non-shockable rhythms (asystole and pulseless electrical activity (PEA)).

The main difference in the treatment of these two groups of arrhythmias is the need for attempted defibrillation in patients with VF/pVT. Other actions, including chest compressions, airway management and ventilation, venous access, injection of adrenaline and the identification and correction of reversible factors, are common to both groups.

The ALS algorithm (Figure 4.1) is a standardised approach to the patient with cardiorespiratory arrest. This has the advantage of enabling treatment to be delivered expediently, without protracted discussion. Each member of the resuscitation team can predict and prepare for the next stage in the patient's treatment, making the team more efficient.

The most important interventions that improve survival after cardiac arrest are early and uninterrupted high quality chest compressions, and early defibrillation for VF/pVT. Although drugs and advanced airways are still included among ALS interventions, there is limited evidence to support their use. Drugs and advanced airways are therefore of secondary importance to high quality, uninterrupted chest compressions and early defibrillation.

Chapter 6 deals with the recognition of cardiac arrest rhythms. If you are not experienced and trained in the recognition of cardiac arrest rhythms use an automated external defibrillator (AED). Some defibrillators have both a manual and AED capability. Once switched on, the AED will give voice and visual prompts that will guide you through the correct sequence of actions.

ILS

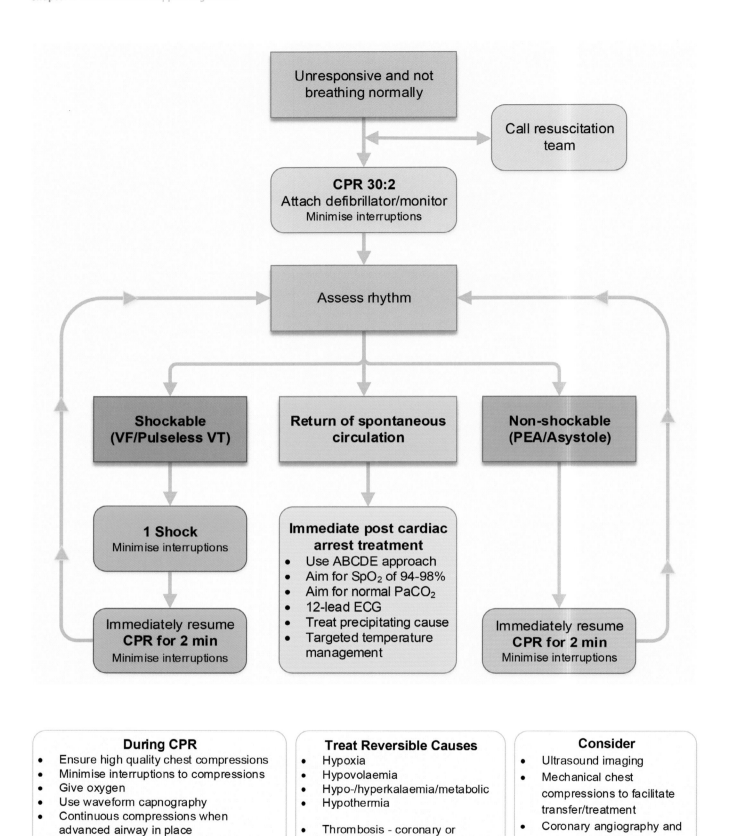

Figure 4.1 Adult Advanced Life Support algorithm

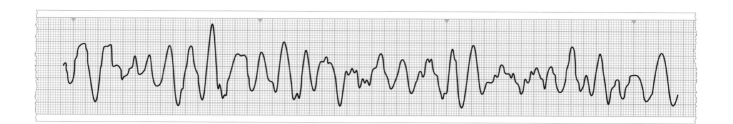

Shockable rhythms (VF/pVT)

The first monitored rhythm is VF/pVT (Figure 4.2) in approximately 20% of cardiac arrests, both in- or out-of-hospital.

Treatment of shockable rhythms (VF/pVT)

A manual defibrillator is used in the sequence described below. Further information about defibrillation can be found in Chapter 7.

1. Confirm cardiac arrest – check for signs of life or if trained to do so, normal breathing and pulse simultaneously.

2. Call the resuscitation team.

3. Give uninterrupted chest compressions while applying self-adhesive defibrillation/monitoring pads – one below the right clavicle and the other in the V6 position in the midaxillary line.

4. Plan actions before pausing CPR for rhythm analysis and communicate these to the team.

5. Stop chest compressions; confirm VF/pVT from the ECG. This pause in chest compressions should be brief and no longer than 5 seconds.

6. Resume chest compressions immediately; warn all rescuers **other than the individual performing the chest compressions** to "stand clear" and remove any oxygen delivery device as appropriate.

7. The designated person selects the appropriate energy on the defibrillator and presses the charge button (Figure 4.3). Choose an energy setting of at least 150 J for the first shock, the same or a higher energy for subsequent shocks, or follow the manufacturer's guidance for the particular defibrillator being used.

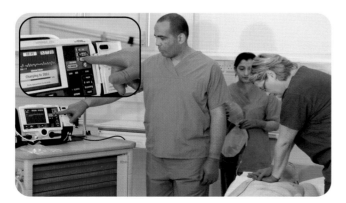

Figure 4.3 Continue chest compressions during defibrillator charging – everyone else stands clear

8. Ensure that the rescuer giving the compressions is the only person touching the patient.

9. Once the defibrillator is charged and the safety check is complete, tell the rescuer doing the chest compressions to "stand clear"; when clear, give the shock (Figure 4.4).

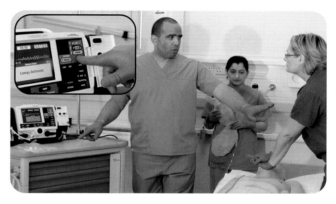

Figure 4.4 Shock delivery – no-one touches the patient when the shock is delivered

10. After shock delivery immediately restart CPR using a ratio of 30:2 (Figure 4.5), starting with chest compressions. Do not pause to reassess the rhythm or feel for a pulse. This pause in chest compressions should be brief and no longer than 5 seconds.

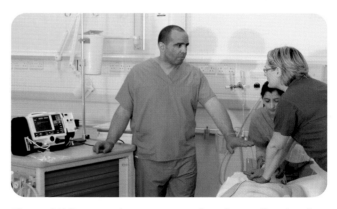

Figure 4.5 Restart chest compressions immediately after shock delivery

11. Continue CPR for 2 minutes; the team leader prepares the team for the next pause in CPR.

12. Pause briefly to check the monitor.

13. If VF/pVT, repeat steps 6–12 above and deliver a second shock.

14. If VF/pVT persists, repeat steps 6–8 above and deliver a third shock. Resume chest compressions immediately. Give adrenaline 1 mg IV and amiodarone 300 mg IV while performing a further 2 minutes CPR. Withhold adrenaline if there are signs of ROSC during CPR.

15. Repeat this 2 minute CPR – rhythm/pulse check – defibrillation sequence if VF/pVT persists.

16. Give further adrenaline 1 mg IV after alternate shocks (i.e. approximately every 3–5 minutes).

17. If organised electrical activity compatible with a cardiac output is seen during a rhythm check, seek evidence of return of spontaneous circulation (ROSC) (check for signs of life, a central pulse, and end-tidal carbon dioxide (CO_2) on waveform capnography if available):

    a. If there is ROSC, start post-resuscitation care.

    b. If there are no signs of ROSC, continue CPR and switch to the non-shockable algorithm.

18. If asystole is seen, continue CPR and switch to the non-shockable algorithm.

Minimise the interval between stopping compressions and delivering a shock. Longer interruptions to chest compressions reduce the chance of a shock restoring a spontaneous circulation.

Chest compressions are resumed immediately after a shock without checking the rhythm or a pulse because even if the defibrillation attempt is successful in restoring a perfusing rhythm, it is very rare for a pulse to be palpable immediately after defibrillation and the delay in trying to palpate a pulse will further compromise the myocardium if a perfusing rhythm has not been restored. If a perfusing rhythm has been restored, giving chest compressions does not increase the chance of VF recurring.

The first dose of adrenaline is given during the 2-minute period of CPR after delivery of the third shock.

Give amiodarone 300 mg after three defibrillation attempts. Do not stop CPR to check the rhythm before giving drugs unless there are clear signs of ROSC.

Subsequent doses of adrenaline are given after alternate 2-minute loops of CPR (which equates to every 3–5 minutes) for as long as cardiac arrest persists. If VF/pVT persists, or recurs, a further dose of 150 mg amiodarone may be given after a total of five defibrillation attempts. Lidocaine, 1 mg kg^{-1}, may be used as an alternative if amiodarone is not available, but do not give lidocaine if amiodarone has been given already.

When the rhythm is checked 2 minutes after giving a shock, if a non-shockable rhythm is present and the rhythm is organised (complexes appear regular or narrow), try to palpate a central pulse and look for other evidence of ROSC (e.g. sudden increase in end-tidal CO_2 or evidence of cardiac output on any invasive monitoring equipment).

Keep rhythm checks brief and undertake pulse checks only if an organised rhythm is observed. If an organised rhythm is seen during a 2-minute period of CPR, do not interrupt chest compressions to palpate a pulse unless the patient shows signs of life suggesting ROSC. If there is any doubt about the presence of a pulse in the presence of an organised rhythm, resume CPR. If the patient has ROSC, begin post-resuscitation care. If the patient's rhythm changes to asystole or PEA, see non-shockable rhythms below.

Do not spend time attempting to distinguish fine VF from coarse VF, or extremely fine VF from asystole during the 5 second rhythm check. If the rhythm appears to be VF give a shock, and if it appears to be asystole continue chest compressions. Avoid excessive interruptions in chest compression for rhythm analysis. Rescuers who are not comfortable with rapid rhythm assessment during CPR should use an automated external defibrillator.

Precordial thump

A precordial thump rarely works for cardioversion of a shockable rhythm so don't use it routinely. Consider a precordial thump when it can be used without delay whilst awaiting the arrival of a defibrillator in a monitored VF/pVT arrest. Using the ulnar edge of a tightly clenched fist, deliver a sharp impact to the lower half of the sternum from a height of about 20 cm, then retract the fist immediately to create an impulse-like stimulus.

Witnessed and monitored VF/pVT cardiac arrest

If a patient has a monitored and witnessed cardiac arrest in the catheter laboratory, coronary care unit, a critical care area, or whilst monitored after cardiac surgery, and a manual defibrillator is rapidly available:

- Confirm cardiac arrest and shout for help.

- If the initial rhythm is VF/pVT, give up to three quick successive (stacked) shocks.

- Rapidly check for a rhythm change and, if appropriate check for a pulse and other signs of ROSC after each defibrillation attempt.

- Start chest compressions and continue CPR for 2 minutes if the third shock is unsuccessful.

This three-shock strategy may also be considered for an initial, witnessed VF/pVT cardiac arrest if the patient is already connected to a manual defibrillator – these circumstances are rare.

If this initial three-shock strategy is unsuccessful for a monitored VF/pVT cardiac arrest, follow the ALS algorithm and treat these three-shocks as if only the first single shock has been given. These initial three stacked shocks are considered as giving the first shock in the ALS algorithm.

Non-shockable rhythms (PEA and asystole)

Pulseless electrical activity (PEA) is cardiac arrest in the presence of electrical activity (other than ventricular tachyarrhythmia) that would normally be associated with a palpable pulse. These patients often have some mechanical myocardial contractions but they are too weak to produce a detectable pulse or blood pressure. PEA may be caused by reversible conditions that can be treated (see below). Survival following cardiac arrest with asystole or PEA is unlikely unless a reversible cause can be found and treated quickly and effectively.

Asystole is the absence of electrical activity on the ECG trace. Make sure the ECG pads are attached to the chest and the correct monitoring mode is selected. Whenever a diagnosis of asystole is made, check the ECG carefully for the presence of P waves because in this situation ventricular standstill may be treated effectively by cardiac pacing. Attempts to pace true asystole are unlikely to be successful.

Treatment for PEA and asystole

- Start CPR 30:2.

- Give adrenaline 1 mg IV/IO as soon as intravascular access is achieved.

- Continue CPR 30:2 until the airway is secured – then continue chest compressions without pausing during ventilation.

- Recheck the rhythm after 2 minutes:
  - If electrical activity compatible with a pulse is seen, check for a pulse and/or signs of life:
    - if a pulse and/or signs of life are present, start post-resuscitation care
    - if no pulse and/or no signs of life are present (PEA or asystole):
      - continue CPR
      - recheck the rhythm after 2 minutes and proceed accordingly
      - give further adrenaline 1 mg IV every 3–5 minutes (during alternate 2-minute loops of CPR)
  - If VF/pVT at rhythm check, change to shockable side of algorithm.

During CPR

During the treatment of persistent VF/pVT or PEA/asystole, emphasis is placed on good quality chest compressions between defibrillation attempts, recognising and treating reversible causes (4 Hs and 4 Ts), obtaining a secure airway, and vascular access.

During CPR with a 30:2 ratio, the underlying rhythm may be seen clearly on the monitor during the pauses for ventilation. If VF is seen during this brief pause (whether on the shockable or non-shockable side of the algorithm), do not attempt defibrillation at this stage; instead, continue with CPR until the 2-minute period is completed. Knowing that the rhythm is VF, the team should be fully prepared to deliver a shock with minimal delay at the end of the 2-minute period of CPR.

Maintain high quality, uninterrupted chest compressions

The quality of chest compressions and ventilations are important determinants of outcome, yet are frequently performed poorly by healthcare professionals. Avoid interruptions in chest compressions. Ensure compressions are of adequate depth (5–6 cm) and rate (100–120 min^{-1}), and ensure there is full recoil of the chest at the end of each compression.

As soon as the airway is secured, continue chest compressions without pausing during ventilation. To reduce fatigue, change the individual undertaking compressions every 2 minute or earlier if necessary.

Airway and ventilation

Use a bag-mask, or preferably, a supraglottic airway (e.g. laryngeal mask airway, i-gel) if no-one on the resuscitation team is skilled in tracheal intubation (Chapter 5). Once a supraglottic airway has been inserted, attempt to deliver continuous chest compressions, uninterrupted during ventilation. Ventilate the lungs at 10 breaths per minute; do not hyperventilate the lungs. If excessive gas leakage causes inadequate ventilation of the patient's lungs, chest compressions will have to be interrupted to enable ventilation (using a compression: ventilation ratio of 30:2).

No studies have shown that tracheal intubation increases survival after cardiac arrest. Tracheal intubation should be attempted only if the healthcare provider is properly trained and has regular, ongoing experience with the technique. Avoid stopping chest compressions during laryngoscopy and intubation; if necessary, a brief pause in chest compressions may be required as the tube is passed between the vocal cords, but this pause should not exceed 5 seconds. Alternatively, to avoid any interruptions in chest compressions, the intubation attempt may be deferred until after ROSC. After intubation, confirm correct tube position with waveform capnography, and secure it adequately. Once the patient's trachea has been intubated, continue chest compressions, at a rate of 100–120 min^{-1} without pausing during ventilation.

Monitoring during CPR

Several methods can be used to monitor the patient during CPR and potentially help guide ALS interventions. These include:

- **Clinical signs** such as breathing efforts, movements and eye opening can occur during CPR. These can indicate ROSC and require verification by a rhythm and pulse check, but can also occur because high quality CPR can generate a sufficient circulation to restore signs of life including consciousness.

- **Pulse checks** can be used to identify ROSC when there is an ECG rhythm compatible with a pulse, but may not detect pulses in those with low cardiac output states and a low blood pressure.

- **Monitoring the heart rhythm** through pads, paddles or ECG electrodes is a standard part of ALS. Motion artefacts prevent reliable heart rhythm assessment during chest compressions.

- **End-tidal CO_2 measured with waveform capnography.** The use of waveform capnography during CPR is addressed in more detail below.

- **Feedback or prompt devices** can monitor CPR quality data such as compression rate and depth during CPR, and provide real-time feedback to rescuers. Be aware that some devices fail to compensate for compression of the underlying mattress during CPR on a bed when providing feedback. The use of these devices should be as part of a broader system of care that includes CPR quality improvement initiatives such as debriefing based on the data collected.

- **Blood sampling and analysis** during CPR can be used to identify potentially reversible causes of cardiac arrest. Avoid finger prick samples because they may not be reliable; instead, use samples from veins or arteries.

- **Invasive cardiovascular monitoring** in critical care settings (e.g. continuous arterial blood pressure and central venous pressure monitoring). Invasive arterial pressure monitoring will enable the detection of even very low blood pressure values when ROSC is achieved.

- The use of **focused echocardiography/ultrasound** to identify and treat reversible causes of cardiac arrest, and identify low cardiac output states ('pseudo-PEA') is discussed below.

Waveform capnography during advanced life support

Carbon dioxide is a waste product of metabolism; approximately 400 L are produced each day. It is carried in the blood to the lungs where it is exhaled. End-tidal CO_2 is the partial pressure of CO_2 at the end of an exhaled breath. It reflects cardiac output and lung blood flow (CO_2 is transported by the venous system to the right side of the heart and then pumped to the lungs by the right ventricle). During CPR, end-tidal CO_2 values are low, reflecting the low cardiac output generated by chest compression. Waveform capnography enables continuous real time end-tidal CO_2 to be monitored during CPR. It works most reliably in patients

who have a tracheal tube, but can also be used with a supraglottic airway or bag-mask.

The role of waveform capnography during CPR

- **Ensuring tracheal tube placement in the trachea.** Correct tube placement also relies on observation and auscultation to ensure both lungs are ventilated.

- **Monitoring ventilation rate during CPR** and avoiding hyperventilation.

- **Monitoring the quality of chest compressions** during CPR. End-tidal CO_2 values are associated with compression depth and ventilation rate and a greater depth of chest compression will increase the value.

- **Identifying ROSC during CPR.** An increase in end-tidal CO_2 during CPR may indicate ROSC, and prevent unnecessary and potentially harmful administration of adrenaline in a patient with ROSC. If ROSC is suspected during CPR withhold adrenaline. Give adrenaline if cardiac arrest is confirmed at the next rhythm check.

- **Prognostication during CPR.** Precise values of end-tidal CO_2 depend on several factors including the cause of cardiac arrest, bystander CPR, chest compression quality, ventilation rate and volume, time from cardiac arrest and the use of adrenaline. Low end-tidal CO_2 values during CPR are associated with lower ROSC rates and increased mortality, and high values with better ROSC and survival. End-tidal CO_2 values should be considered only as part of a multi-modal approach to decision-making for prognostication during CPR.

Vascular access

The role of drugs during cardiac arrest is uncertain. Some patients will already have intravenous access before they have a cardiac arrest. If this is not the case ensure CPR has started and defibrillation, if appropriate, attempted before considering vascular access.

Insertion of a central venous catheter requires interruption of CPR and is associated with several potential complications. Peripheral venous cannulation is quicker, easier, and safer. Drugs injected peripherally must be followed by a flush of at least 20 mL of fluid and elevation of the extremity for 10–20 seconds to facilitate drug delivery to the central circulation.

If intravenous access cannot be established within the first few minutes of resuscitation, consider gaining intraosseous (IO) access (Figure 4.6). The three main insertion sites for IO access for use during CPR in adults are the proximal humerus, proximal tibia and distal tibia. Learn to use the IO device that you have in your hospital. Once IO access has been confirmed, resuscitation drugs including adrenaline and amiodarone can be infused. Fluids and blood products can also be delivered but pressure will be needed to achieve reasonable flow rates using either a pressure bag or a syringe.

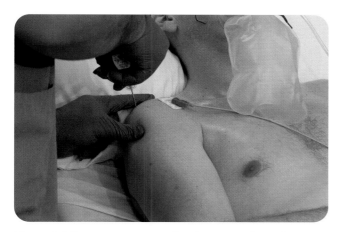

Figure 4.6 Intraosseous needle placement into the humerus

Identification and treatment of reversible causes

Potential causes or aggravating factors for which specific treatment exists must be considered during any cardiac arrest. For ease of memory, these are divided into two groups of four based upon their initial letter – either H or T (Figure 4.7).

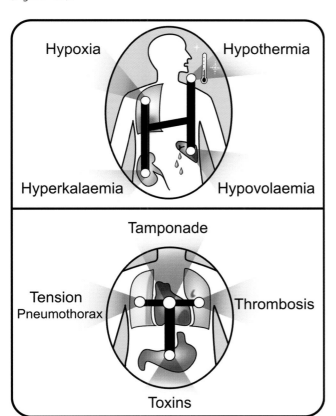

Figure 4.7 The four Hs and four Ts

- Hypoxia

- Hypovolaemia

- Hyperkalaemia, hypokalaemia, hypoglycaemia, hypocalcaemia, acidaemia and other metabolic disorders

- Hypothermia

- Thrombosis (coronary or pulmonary)

- Tension pneumothorax

- Tamponade – cardiac

- Toxins

The four Hs

Minimise the risk of hypoxia by ensuring that the patient's lungs are ventilated adequately with 100% oxygen during CPR. Check carefully that the tracheal tube is not misplaced in a bronchus or the oesophagus.

Pulseless electrical activity caused by hypovolaemia is usually due to severe bleeding such as might be caused by trauma, gastrointestinal bleeding, or rupture of an aortic aneurysm. Restore intravascular volume rapidly with fluid and blood. Obviously, such patients need urgent control of bleeding by surgery or other means (e.g. compression, interventional radiology, tourniquet).

Hyperkalaemia, hypokalaemia, hypoglycaemia, hypocalcaemia, acidaemia and other metabolic disorders are detected by biochemical tests or suggested by the patient's medical history (e.g. renal failure). A 12-lead ECG may help diagnosis. Intravenous calcium chloride is indicated in the presence of hyperkalaemia, hypocalcaemia, and calcium channel-blocker overdose. Always measure the blood glucose to exclude hypoglycaemia.

Consider hypothermia; use a low reading thermometer.

The four Ts

Coronary thrombosis is a common cause of cardiac arrest. If initial resuscitation with advanced life support measures is not successful in some specialist hospitals, it is feasible to perform percutaneous coronary angiography and percutaneous coronary intervention during ongoing CPR. This usually requires an automated mechanical chest compression device or heart-bypass type machine (extra-corporeal life support) to maintain a circulation during the procedure.

The commonest cause of thromboembolic or mechanical circulatory obstruction is massive pulmonary embolism. If pulmonary embolism is thought to be the cause of cardiac arrest, consider giving a thrombolytic drug immediately.

A tension pneumothorax can cause PEA. The diagnosis is made clinically. Signs of tension pneumothorax include: decreased air entry, decreased expansion and hyper-resonance to percussion on the affected side; tracheal deviation away from the affected side. Decompress rapidly by thoracostomy or needle thoracocentesis and then insert a chest drain.

Cardiac tamponade is difficult to diagnose because the typical signs of distended neck veins and hypotension cannot be assessed during cardiac arrest. Cardiac arrest after penetrating chest trauma or after cardiac surgery should raise strong suspicion of tamponade – the need for needle pericardiocentesis or resuscitative thoracotomy should be considered.

If there is no specific history of accidental or deliberate ingestion, poisoning by therapeutic or toxic substances is difficult to detect and may only be shown by laboratory investigations. Where available, the appropriate antidotes should be used, but most often treatment is supportive.

Ultrasound for monitoring and detection of reversible causes during CPR

In skilled hands, focused echocardiography/ultrasound can detect potentially reversible causes of cardiac arrest (e.g. cardiac tamponade, pulmonary embolism, ischaemia (regional wall motion abnormality), aortic dissection, hypovolaemia, pneumothorax). This requires special training to ensure that interruptions to chest compressions are to be minimised to less than 10 seconds.

Signs of life

If signs of life (such as regular respiratory effort, movement) or readings from patient monitors compatible with ROSC (e.g. sudden increase in end-tidal carbon dioxide or arterial blood pressure waveform) appear during CPR, stop CPR briefly and check the monitor. If an organised rhythm is present, check for a pulse. If a pulse is palpable, continue post-resuscitation care. If no pulse is present, continue CPR.

The duration of a resuscitation attempt

If attempts at obtaining ROSC are unsuccessful the resuscitation team leader should discuss stopping CPR with the team. The decision to stop CPR requires clinical judgement and a careful assessment of the likelihood of achieving ROSC. If it was considered appropriate to start resuscitation, it is usually considered worthwhile continuing, as long as the patient remains in VF/pVT, or there is a potentially reversible cause that can be treated.

Diagnosing death after unsuccessful resuscitation

If CPR does not achieve ROSC and a decision is made to discontinue CPR efforts, after stopping CPR observe the patient for a minimum of 5 minutes before confirming death. The absence of mechanical cardiac function is normally confirmed using a combination of the following:

- absence of a central pulse on palpation

- absence of heart sounds on auscultation.

One or more of the following can supplement these criteria:

- asystole on a continuous ECG display

- absence of pulsatile flow using direct intra-arterial pressure monitoring

- absence of contractile activity using echocardiography.

Any return of cardiac or respiratory activity during this period of observation should prompt a further 5 minutes observation from the cardiorespiratory arrest. After 5 minutes of continued cardiorespiratory arrest, the absence of pupillary responses to light, corneal reflexes, and motor response to supra-orbital pressure should be confirmed. The time of death is recorded as the time at which these criteria are fulfilled.

Post-event tasks

At the end of the resuscitation attempt further tasks include:

1. Ongoing care of the patient, and allocation of further team roles and responsibilities including handover to other teams.

2. Documentation of the resuscitation attempt. Use information from defibrillators and monitors to help document events and times.

3. Communication with relatives.

4. An immediate post-event debriefing ('Hot' debriefing). This is normally led by the resuscitation team leader, focuses on immediate issues and concerns, and is usually of short duration. This can be difficult if the patient has ROSC, as focus then inevitably shifts to post-resuscitation care. A delayed facilitated debriefing ('Cold' debriefing) is also useful.

5. Ensuring equipment and drug trolleys are replenished.

6. Ensuring audit forms are completed.

Summary learning

- **The ALS algorithm provides a framework for the standardised resuscitation of all adult patients in cardiac arrest.**
- **The delivery of high quality chest compression with minimal interruptions is an important determinant of outcome.**
- **Treatment depends on the underlying rhythm.**
- **Look for reversible causes and, if present, treat early.**
- **Secure the airway early to enable continuous chest compressions.**
- **Use waveform capnography to help assess and guide resuscitation interventions.**

My key take-home messages from this chapter

Further reading

Academy of Medical Royal Colleges. A code of practice for the diagnosis and confirmation of death. 2008. http://www.aomrc.org.uk

Cook TM, Woodall N, Harper J, Benger J; Fourth National Audit Project. Major complications of airway management in the UK: results of the Fourth National Audit Project of the Royal College of Anaesthetists and the Difficult Airway Society. Part 2: intensive care and emergency departments. Br J Anaesth. 2011;106:632-42.

Couper K, Kimani PK, Abella BS, et al. The System-Wide Effect of Real-Time Audiovisual Feedback and Postevent Debriefing for In-Hospital Cardiac Arrest: The Cardiopulmonary Resuscitation Quality Improvement Initiative. Crit Care Med. 2015 Jul 16. doi: 10.1097/CCM.0000000000001202.

Diagnosis of death after cessation of cardiopulmonary resuscitation. Signal 1329. National Reporting and Learning System (NRLS) and National Patient Safety Agency (NPSA). February 2012.

FEEL – Focused Echocardiography in Emergency Life Support. https://www.resus.org.uk/information-on-courses/focused-echocardiography-in-emergency-life-support/

Gates S, Quinn T, Deakin CD, Blair L, Couper K, Perkins GD. Mechanical chest compression for out of hospital cardiac arrest: Systematic review and meta-analysis. Resuscitation 2015;94:91–7.

Nolan JP, Soar J, Smith GB, et al. Incidence and outcome of in-hospital cardiac arrest in the United Kingdom National Cardiac Arrest Audit. Resuscitation 2014;85:987-92.

Soar J, Callaway CW, Aibiki M, et al. Part 4: Advanced life support: 2015 International Consensus on Cardiopulmonary Resuscitation and Emergency Cardiovascular Care Science With Treatment Recommendations. Resuscitation 2015;95:e71-e122.

Soar J, Nolan JP, Bottiger BW, et al. European Resuscitation Council Guidelines for Resuscitation 2015 Section 3 Adult Advanced Life Support. Resuscitation 2015;95:99-146.

ILS

Airway management and ventilation

Contents

- Causes and recognition of airway obstruction
- Techniques for airway management when starting resuscitation
- The use of simple adjuncts to maintain airway patency
- Techniques for ventilating the lungs

Learning outcomes

To enable you to:
- Recognise the causes of airway obstruction
- Recognise and treat choking
- Use basic airway opening techniques
- Understand the role of the pocket mask and bag-mask ventilation
- Understand the role of supraglottic airways

Introduction

Patients requiring resuscitation often have an obstructed airway, usually caused by loss of consciousness, but occasionally obstruction is the primary cause of cardiorespiratory arrest. Prompt assessment, airway opening, and ventilation are essential to help prevent secondary hypoxic damage to the brain and other vital organs. Without adequate oxygenation an arrested heart may not restart.

The airway and ventilation technique used will depend on the patient's condition, the skills of the rescuer and the equipment available. Most patients who have a cardiac arrest will have more than one airway and ventilation technique used during their resuscitation.

Causes of airway obstruction

Obstruction may be partial or complete. It may occur at any level from the nose and mouth down to the level of the trachea and bronchi. In the unconscious patient, the commonest site of airway obstruction is the pharynx – more often at the soft palate and epiglottis rather than the tongue. Obstruction can also be caused by vomit or blood, by regurgitation of gastric contents, by trauma to the airway, or by foreign bodies. Laryngeal obstruction can be because of oedema caused by burns, inflammation or anaphylaxis. Upper airway stimulation, or an inhaled foreign body, can cause laryngeal spasm (laryngospasm). Obstruction of the airway below the larynx is less common, but may be caused by excessive bronchial secretions, mucosal oedema, bronchospasm, pulmonary oedema, or aspiration of gastric contents. Extrinsic compression of the airway may also occur above or below the larynx (e.g. trauma, haematoma or tumour).

ILS

Recognition of airway obstruction

Recognition is best achieved by the look, listen and feel approach:

- LOOK for chest and abdominal movements

- LISTEN and FEEL for airflow at the mouth and nose.

In partial airway obstruction, air entry is diminished and usually noisy:

- Inspiratory stridor is caused by obstruction at the larynx or above.

- Expiratory wheeze suggests obstruction of the lower airways, which tend to collapse and obstruct during expiration.

- Gurgling suggests there is liquid or semisolid material in the upper airways.

- Snoring arises when the pharynx is partially occluded by the tongue or palate.

- Crowing or stridor is the sound of laryngeal spasm or obstruction.

During normal breathing, the abdomen is pushed out as the chest wall expands. In contrast, if the airway is obstructed the abdomen is seen to be pushed out as the chest is drawn in during attempts to inspire. This is often described as 'see-saw breathing'. If the airway is obstructed, accessory muscles of respiration are used: the neck and shoulder muscles contract to assist movement of the thoracic cage. There may also be intercostal and subcostal recession. Full examination of the neck, chest and abdomen is needed to differentiate these paradoxical movements from normal breathing; it is sometimes very difficult and you must listen for the absence of breath sounds to diagnose complete airway obstruction. When listening, remember that normal breathing should be quiet; obstructed breathing will be silent; but noisy breathing indicates partial airway obstruction. Unless obstruction is relieved to allow adequate ventilation within a very few minutes, neurological and other vital organ injury will occur, leading to cardiac arrest.

Whenever possible, give high-concentration oxygen during the attempt to relieve airway obstruction. Arterial blood oxygen saturation (SaO_2) measurements (normally using pulse oximetry (SpO_2)) will guide further use of oxygen as airway patency improves. If airway patency remains poor and SaO_2 remains low, continue to give high-concentration oxygen. As airway patency improves, blood oxygen saturation values will be restored more rapidly if the inspired oxygen concentration is initially high. Inspired oxygen concentrations can then be adjusted to maintain an SpO_2 at 94–98%.

Choking

Recognition of choking

Foreign bodies may cause either mild or severe airway obstruction. The signs and symptoms enabling differentiation between mild and severe airway obstruction are summarised in Table 5.1.

General signs of choking	
• Attack occurs while eating • Patient may clutch his neck	
Signs of severe airway obstruction	**Signs of mild airway obstruction**
Response to question 'Are you choking?' • Patient unable to speak • Patient may respond by nodding	*Response to question 'Are you choking?'* • Patient speaks and answers yes
Other signs • Patient unable to breathe • Breathing sounds wheezy • Attempts at coughing are silent • Patient may be unconscious	*Other signs* • Patient is able to speak, cough, and breathe

Table 5.1 Signs of choking

Treatment of adult choking

1. If the patient shows signs of mild airway obstruction (Figure 5.1):

   - Encourage him to continue coughing, but do nothing else.

2. If the patient shows signs of severe airway obstruction and is conscious:

   - Give up to 5 back blows.

     - Stand to the side and slightly behind the patient.

     - Support the chest with one hand and lean the patient well forwards.

     - Give up to 5 sharp blows between the scapulae with the heel of the other hand.

   - Check to see if each back blow has relieved the airway obstruction.

   - If 5 back blows fail to relieve the airway obstruction give up to 5 abdominal thrusts.

     - Stand behind the patient and put both arms round the upper part of his abdomen.

     - Place a clenched fist just under the xiphisternum; grasp this hand with your other hand and pull sharply inwards and upwards.

     - Repeat up to 5 times.

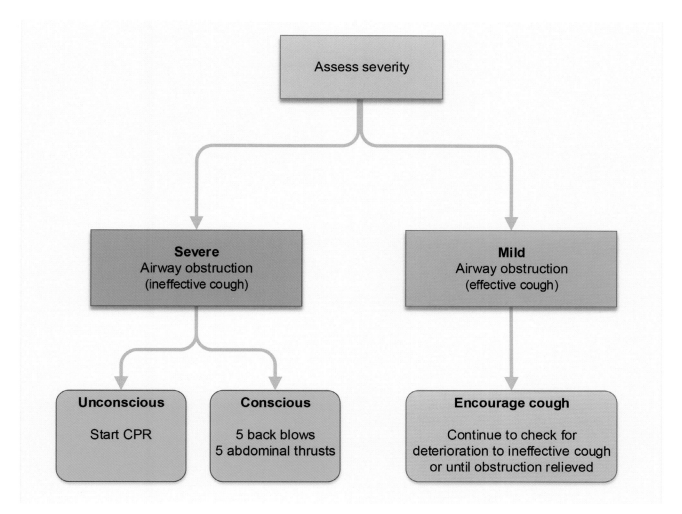

Figure 5.1 Adult choking algorithm

- If the obstruction is still not relieved, continue alternating 5 back blows with abdominal thrusts.

3. If the patient becomes unconscious, call the resuscitation team and start CPR.

4. As soon as an individual with appropriate skills is present, look with a laryngoscope and attempt to remove any foreign body with Magill's forceps.

Basic techniques for opening the airway

Once airway obstruction is recognised, take immediate action to relieve the obstruction and maintain a clear airway. Three manoeuvres can be used to relieve upper airway obstruction:

- head tilt
- chin lift
- jaw thrust

Head tilt and chin lift

Place one hand on the patient's forehead and tilt the head back gently; place the fingertips of the other hand under the point of the patient's chin, and gently lift to stretch the anterior neck structures (Figure 5.2).

Jaw thrust

Jaw thrust is another manoeuvre for bringing the mandible forward and relieving obstruction (Figure 5.3). It is most successful when applied with a head tilt.

Technique for jaw thrust

- Identify the angle of the mandible.

- Apply steady upward and forward (anterior) pressure with the index and other fingers placed behind the angle of the mandible.

- Use the thumbs to open the mouth slightly by downward displacement of the chin.

Jaw thrust, or head tilt and chin lift, will usually clear the airway when obstruction is from relaxation of the soft tissues. Check for success by using the look, listen and feel sequence described above. If the airway is still obstructed, look and remove any solid foreign body in the mouth with forceps or suction. Remove broken or displaced dentures but leave well-fitting dentures in place, as they help to maintain the contours of the mouth, which improves the seal for ventilation by mouth-to-mask or bag-mask techniques.

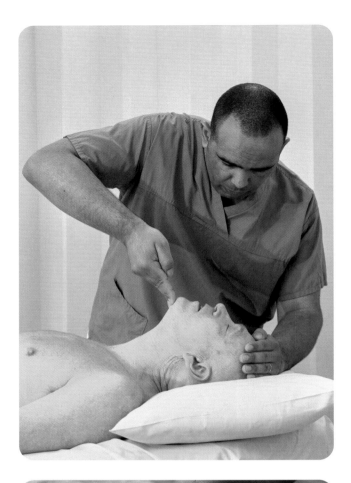

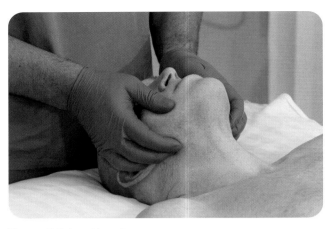

Figure 5.3 Jaw thrust

Airway manoeuvres in a patient with suspected cervical spine injury

If spinal injury is suspected (e.g. if the victim has fallen, been struck on the head or neck, or has been rescued after diving into shallow water) maintain the head, neck, chest, and lumbar region in the neutral position during resuscitation. Excessive head tilt could worsen the injury and damage the cervical spinal cord; however, this complication remains theoretical and the relative risk is unknown. When there is a risk of cervical spine injury, establish a clear upper airway by using jaw thrust or chin lift in combination with manual in-line stabilisation of the head and neck by an assistant. If life-threatening airway obstruction persists despite jaw thrust or chin lift, add head tilt a small amount at a time until the airway is open; establishing airway and breathing takes priority over concerns about a potential cervical spine injury.

Adjuncts to basic airway techniques

Simple airway adjuncts are often helpful, and sometimes essential to maintain an open airway, particularly when resuscitation is prolonged. Oropharyngeal and nasopharyngeal airways overcome soft palate obstruction and backward tongue displacement in an unconscious patient, but head tilt and jaw thrust may also be necessary.

Oropharyngeal airway

The oropharyngeal (Guedel) airway is a curved plastic tube, flanged and reinforced at the oral end and flattened to fit neatly between the tongue and hard palate (Figure 5.4). There are sizes suitable for small and large adults. Estimate the size by selecting an airway with a length equal to the vertical distance between the patient's incisors and the angle of the jaw (Figure 5.5). The most common sizes are 2 for small, 3 for medium and 4 for large adults. An airway that is slightly too big will be more beneficial than one that is slightly too small.

Oropharyngeal airways are intended only for unconscious patients; attempted insertion in semi-comatose patients may provoke vomiting or laryngospasm. If a patient is intolerant of an oral airway, they do not need one.

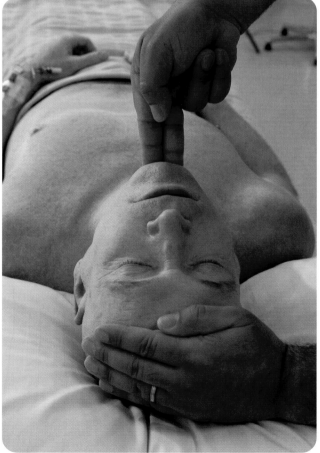

Figure 5.2 Head tilt and chin lift

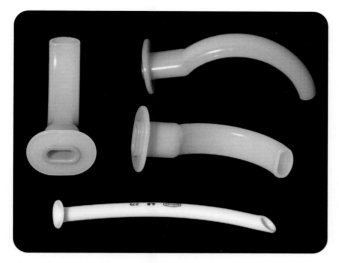

Figure 5.4 Oropharyngeal and nasopharyngeal airways

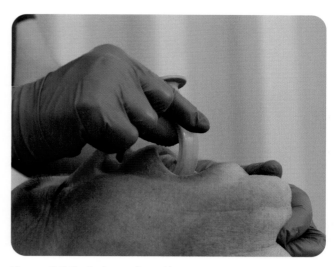

Figure 5.6 Oral airway insertion

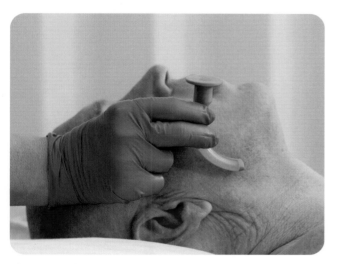

Figure 5.5 Sizing an oropharyngeal airway

Technique for insertion of an oropharyngeal airway

- Open the patient's mouth and ensure that there is nothing in the mouth that could be pushed into the larynx; use suction if necessary.

- Introduce the airway past the teeth or gums 'upside-down' and then rotate it through 180° as it passes beyond the hard palate and into the oropharynx (Figure 5.6). This manoeuvre lessens the chance of pushing the tongue backwards and downwards. Be careful not to lever the front incisors. The patient must be sufficiently obtunded not to gag or strain. If any reflex responses are seen, remove the airway. If placement is correct, obstruction will be relieved and the flattened reinforced section will fit neatly between the patient's front teeth or gums.

- After insertion, check the airway by the look, listen and feel approach, while maintaining alignment of the head and neck with head tilt, chin lift or jaw thrust as necessary.

Nasopharyngeal airway

This is made from soft malleable plastic, bevelled at one end and with a flange at the other (Figure 5.4). In patients who are not deeply unconscious, it is tolerated better than an oropharyngeal airway. It may be life-saving in patients with clenched jaws, trismus or maxillofacial injuries. Use with caution in patients with a suspected fracture of the base of skull, and remember they often cause bleeding inside the nose.

The tubes are sized in millimetres according to their internal diameter, and the length increases with diameter. Sizes 6-7 mm are suitable for adults. If the tube is too long it may stimulate the laryngeal or glossopharyngeal reflexes and cause laryngospasm or vomiting. Traditional methods of sizing a nasopharyngeal airway (measurement against the patient's little finger or anterior nares) are unreliable.

Be careful if you use a nasopharyngeal airway. About 30% of patients get a nose bleed, and if the tube is too long it can make the patient gag and vomit.

Technique for insertion of a nasopharyngeal airway

- Some older designs require a safety pin to be inserted through the flange as an extra precaution against the airway disappearing into the nose. Insert the safety pin with care before inserting the airway.

- Lubricate the airway thoroughly using water-soluble jelly.

- Insert the airway bevel end first, vertically along the floor of the nose with a slight twisting action (Figure 5.7). Try the right nostril first. If any obstruction is met, try the left nostril.

- Once in place, check for patency and ventilation by look, listen, and feel, and if necessary maintain correct alignment of the head and neck with chin lift or jaw thrust techniques.

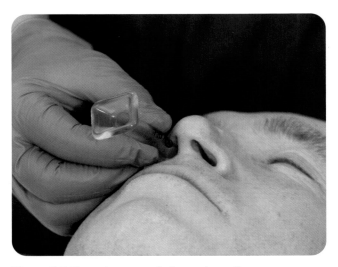

Figure 5.7 Nasopharyngeal airway insertion

Oxygen

Ventilate the lungs with 100% oxygen until return of spontaneous circulation (ROSC) is achieved. After ROSC is achieved and in any acutely ill, or unconscious patient, give high-flow oxygen until the oxygen saturation of arterial blood (SaO$_2$) can be measured reliably with pulse oximetry (SpO$_2$). A low blood oxygen level (hypoxaemia) is harmful, and after ROSC a high blood oxygen level (hyperoxaemia) could be harmful. A standard oxygen mask (e.g. Hudson mask) will deliver up to 50% inspired oxygen, providing the flow of oxygen is high enough. Initially, give the highest possible oxygen concentration – a mask with a reservoir bag (non-rebreathing mask) can deliver an inspired oxygen concentration of 85% at flows of 10–15 L min^{-1}. Monitor the oxygen saturation by pulse oximeter (SpO$_2$) or arterial blood gases to enable titration of the inspired oxygen concentration. When blood oxygen saturation can be measured reliably, oxygen saturations should be maintained between 94–98%; or between 88–92% if the patient has chronic obstructive pulmonary disease (COPD).

Suction

Use a wide-bore rigid sucker (Yankauer) to remove liquid (blood, saliva and gastric contents) from the upper airway (Figure 5.8). Be careful if the patient has an intact gag reflex – suction can provoke vomiting. Fine-bore flexible suction catheters can be used in patients with limited mouth opening. They can also be passed through oropharyngeal or nasopharyngeal airways. Make sure you know how to use any portable suction equipment in your clinical area. Thick vomit can be difficult to suction without a large bore sucker and good suction. Large chunks of food may have to be removed by hand or Magill's forceps.

Ventilation

Patients with no or inadequate breathing require artificial ventilation. Expired air ventilation (rescue breathing with mouth-to-mouth or mouth-to-mask breaths) is effective but the rescuer's expired oxygen concentration is only 16–17%; so it must be replaced as soon as possible by ventilation with oxygen-enriched air. Mouth-to-mouth

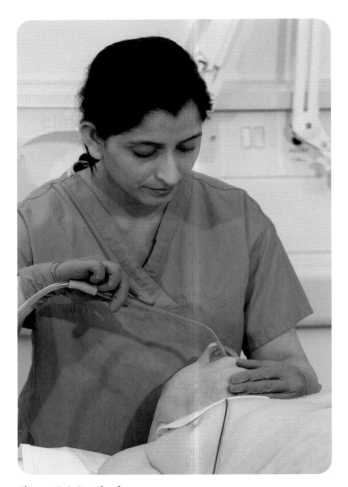

Figure 5.8 Suctioning

ventilation does not require any equipment but is unpleasant, particularly when vomit or blood is present. There are simple adjuncts for avoiding direct person-to-person contact.

Pocket mask

The pocket resuscitation mask is used widely. This is similar to an anaesthetic face mask and enables mouth-to-mask ventilation. It has a unidirectional valve to direct the patient's expired air away from the rescuer. The masks are transparent to allow vomit or blood to be seen. Some masks have a port for oxygen. This port also has a simple one-way flap-valve so there is no leak if oxygen is not attached. When using masks without an oxygen port, supplemental oxygen can be given by placing oxygen tubing underneath one side of the mask and ensuring an adequate seal. The main difficulty is maintaining an airtight seal between the mask and the face, so a two-hand technique is much better (Figure 5.9).

The risks of gastric inflation and subsequent regurgitation are increased by:

- Blowing too hard because of misalignment of the head and neck obstructing the airway and/or tidal volumes that are too large.

- The incompetent oesophageal sphincter of all patients in cardiac arrest.

Give each breath over 1 second, giving a volume that corresponds to visible chest movement; this is a compromise between giving enough volume, minimising the risk of gastric inflation, and allowing enough time for chest compressions. Give 2 ventilations after every 30 chest compressions.

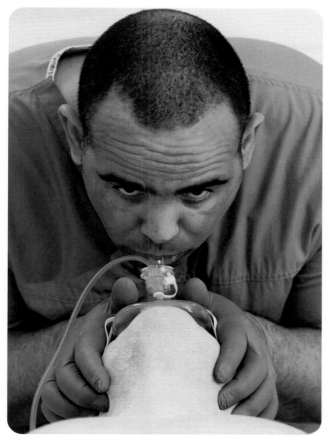

Figure 5.9 Mouth-to-mask ventilation

Technique for mouth-to-mask ventilation

- Place the patient supine with the head in a 'sniffing' position (i.e. neck slightly flexed on a pillow with the head extended (tilted backwards) on the neck).

- Apply the mask to the patient's face using the thumbs of both hands.

- Lift the jaw into the mask with the remaining fingers by exerting pressure behind the angles of the jaw (jaw thrust). At the same time, press the mask onto the face with the thumbs to make a tight seal (Figure 5.9).

- Blow through the inspiratory valve and watch the chest rise.

- Stop inflation and watch the chest fall.

- Reduce any leaks between the face and mask by adjusting the contact pressure, altering the position of the fingers and thumbs, or increasing jaw thrust.

- If oxygen is available, add via the port at a flow of 10 L min⁻¹.

Self-inflating bag

The self-inflating bag can be connected to a face mask (bag-mask), supraglottic airway (e.g. laryngeal mask airway, i-gel) or a tracheal tube. As the bag is squeezed, the contents are delivered to the patient's lungs. On release, the expired gas is diverted to the atmosphere via a one-way valve; the bag then refills automatically via an inlet at the opposite end. When used without supplemental oxygen, the self-inflating bag ventilates the patient's lungs with ambient air only (oxygen concentration 21%). This is increased to around 45% by attaching high-flow oxygen directly to the bag adjacent to the air intake. An inspired oxygen concentration of approximately 85% is achieved if a reservoir system is attached and the oxygen flow is high (10–15 L min⁻¹).

A self-inflating bag enables ventilation with high concentrations of oxygen, but its use requires skill. When used with a face mask, it is difficult to achieve a gas-tight seal while simultaneously performing a jaw thrust with one hand and squeezing the bag with the other. It is easy to hypoventilate because of a leak, or to push down too hard and obstruct the airway. Excessive compression of the bag when used with a face mask can inflate the stomach, further reducing ventilation and greatly increasing the risk of regurgitation and aspiration.

Bag-mask ventilation is better with two people (Figure 5.10). One person holds the face mask in place, using both hands and a jaw thrust, and the other squeezes the bag. The seal will be better and the ventilation will be more effective and safer.

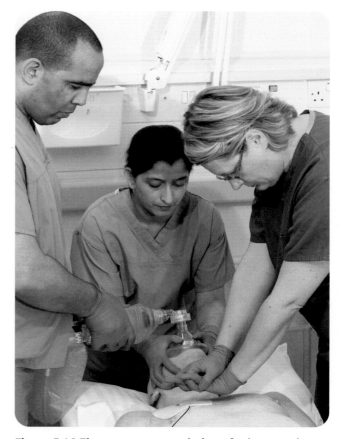

Figure 5.10 The two-person technique for bag-mask ventilation during CPR

Supraglottic airways during CPR

In comparison with bag-mask ventilation, use of supraglottic airways (e.g. laryngeal mask airway, i-gel) may enable more effective ventilation and reduce the risk of gastric inflation. Supraglottic airways sit above the larynx and are easier to insert than a tracheal tube. They can generally be inserted without having to stop chest compressions.

Laryngeal mask airway

The laryngeal mask airway (LMA) is a wide-bore tube with an elliptical inflated cuff, which sits above the laryngeal opening (Figure 5.11). It was introduced into anaesthetic practice in the middle of the 1980s and is a reliable, safe device that can be inserted easily with a high success rate after a short period of training. The LMA does not guarantee protection of the airway, but pulmonary aspiration is uncommon. Provided tidal volumes do not generate high inflation pressures during intermittent positive pressure ventilation (> 20 cm H_2O), gastric inflation is unlikely. Inserting an LMA does not require vigorous movements to align the head and neck, so could be the best adjunct if cervical spine injury is suspected. The LMA is reliable in use during resuscitation by nursing, paramedical and medical staff. As with tracheal intubation, the patient must be deeply unconscious. The LMA is particularly useful if attempted intubation by skilled personnel has failed and bag-mask ventilation is impossible (the 'cannot ventilate, cannot intubate' scenario). The conventional LMA (LMA Classic™) can be sterilised and reused up to 40 times. Many single-use versions are now available and these are more practical for resuscitation use. Many of the single-use LMAs are of a slightly different design and material to the LMA Classic™ and their performance has not been validated during CPR. Modifications of the LMA are also available. The ProSeal LMA (PLMA) is a modified version of the original LMA. A disposable form of the PLMA – the LMA Supreme is more appropriate then the reusable version for use during CPR as it can form an improved seal and has a gastric drainage channel.

Technique for insertion of a laryngeal mask airway

- Try to insert the LMA without stopping chest compressions. If necessary try to limit any pause in chest compressions to a maximum of 5 seconds.

- Choose a LMA of appropriate size. A size 5 will be correct for most men and a size 4 for most women.

- Apply lubricating jelly to the outer face of the cuff area (the part that will not be in contact with the larynx).

- Holding the LMA like a pen, insert it into the mouth (Figure 5.12). Advance the tip with the upper surface applied to the palate until it reaches the posterior pharyngeal wall. Press the mask backwards and downwards around the corner of the pharynx until a resistance is felt as it locates in the back of the pharynx. A slight 45-degree twist will often aid placement if initial attempts at insertion beyond the pharynx are proving difficult.

- Connect the inflating syringe and inflate the cuff with air (a maximum of 40 mL for a size 5 LMA and 30 mL for a size 4 LMA). Do not hold the LMA during inflation. The tube should lift slightly out of the mouth as the cuff finds its correct position.

- If the LMA cannot be inserted within 30 seconds, oxygenate the patient using a pocket mask or bag-mask before reattempting LMA insertion.

- Confirm a clear airway by listening over the chest during inflation and seeing bilateral chest movement. A large, audible leak suggests malposition of the LMA. A small leak is acceptable if chest rise is adequate.

- Secure the LMA with a bandage or tape.

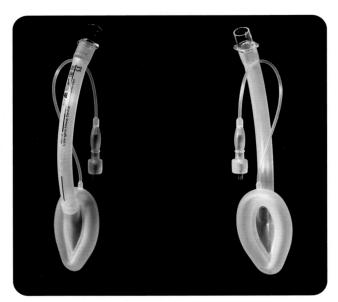

Figure 5.11 Laryngeal mask airway

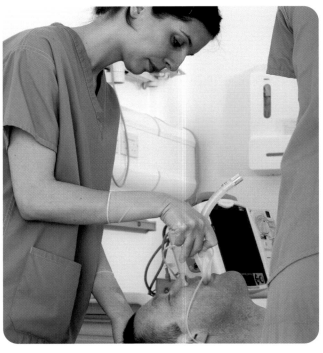

Figure 5.12 Insertion of laryngeal mask airway

Limitations of the laryngeal mask airway

- If there is high airway resistance or the lungs are stiff (pulmonary oedema, bronchospasm, chronic obstructive pulmonary disease) there is a risk of a large leak around the cuff causing hypoventilation. Most of the leak usually escapes through the patient's mouth but some may be forced into the stomach.

- Uninterrupted chest compressions are likely to cause at least some gas leak from the LMA cuff when ventilation is attempted. Attempt continuous compressions initially but abandon this if persistent leaks and hypoventilation occur.

- There is a theoretical risk of aspiration of stomach contents because the LMA does not sit within the larynx like a tracheal tube; however, this is not common in clinical practice.

- If a good airway is not achieved, withdraw the LMA, deflate the cuff and make a new attempt at insertion, ensuring a good alignment of the head and neck and strict adherence to the correct insertion technique.

- Proficiency with the LMA requires practice on patients, which should be gained under the supervision of an anaesthetist in appropriate circumstances.

i-gel airway

The i-gel has a cuff made of jelly-like material and does not require inflation. The stem of the i-gel incorporates a bite block and a narrow oesophageal drain tube that allows a gastric tube to be passed through it (Figure 5.13). It is easy to insert without stopping CPR, requires only minimal training and forms a good laryngeal seal (Figure 5.14). The ease of insertion of the i-gel and its favourable leak pressure make it very attractive as a resuscitation airway device for those inexperienced in tracheal intubation. Use of the i-gel during cardiac arrest has now been reported extensively and it is in widespread use in the UK for both in-hospital and out-of-hospital cardiac arrest.

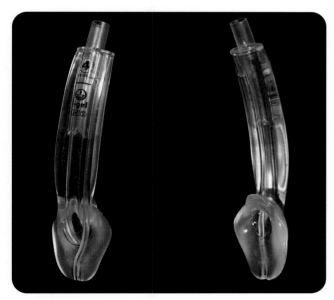

Figure 5.13 i-gel

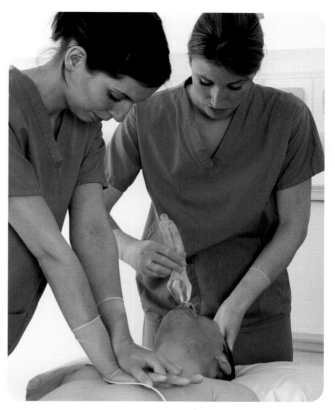

Figure 5.14 Insertion of an i-gel during CPR

Technique for insertion of an i-gel

- Try to maintain chest compressions throughout the insertion attempt; if it is necessary to stop chest compressions during the insertion attempt, limit this pause in chest compressions to a maximum of 5 seconds.

- Select an appropriately sized i-gel: a size 4 will function well in most adults although small females may require a size 3 and tall men a size 5.

- Lubricate the back, sides and front of the i-gel cuff with a thin layer of lubricant

- Grasp the lubricated i-gel firmly along the integral bite block. Position the device so that the i-gel cuff outlet is facing towards the chin of the patient.

- Ensure the patient is in the 'sniffing the morning air' position with head extended and neck flexed. Gently press the chin down before inserting the i-gel.

- Introduce the leading soft tip into the mouth of the patient in a direction towards the hard palate (Figure 5.14).

- Do not apply excessive force to the device during insertion. It is not normally necessary to insert fingers or thumbs into the patient's mouth when inserting the i-gel. If there is early resistance during insertion, get an assistant to apply a jaw thrust or rotate the i-gel.

- Glide the i-gel downwards and backwards along the hard palate with a continuous but gentle push until a definitive resistance is felt.

- At this point the tip of the airway should be located at the upper oesophageal opening and the cuff should be located against the larynx. The incisors should be resting on the integral bite-block.

- A horizontal line at the middle of the integral bite-block represents the approximate position of the teeth when the i-gel is positioned correctly. However, this line is only a guide – there is considerable variation in its location relative to the incisors. In short patients, this line may be at least 1 cm higher then the teeth, even when correctly positioned. In tall patients, the line may not be visible above the teeth.

Patients with tracheostomies or permanent tracheal stomas

A patient with a tracheostomy tube or a permanent tracheal stoma (usually following a laryngectomy) can develop airway obstruction from blockage of the tracheostomy tube or stoma – airway obstruction cannot occur at the level of the pharynx in these patients. Remove any obvious foreign material from the stoma or tracheostomy tube.

When dealing with an emergency it is important to know whether the patient has a normal upper airway and a tracheostomy tube, or has had a laryngectomy:

- Some tracheal tubes can be unblocked by removing an inner tube. Otherwise, if a tracheostomy tube is blocked, remove it and ventilate the patient's lungs by sealing the stoma (the hole at the front of the neck through which the tracheostomy was inserted). The patient will usually have a normal upper airway. Use the standard airway and ventilation techniques outlined in this chapter (e.g. bag-mask ventilation) with the stoma occluded by an airtight dressing. Alternatively, if you are trained to do so replace the tracheostomy tube.

- A laryngectomee is a patient who has had his larynx (voice box) removed, usually for cancer – in lay terms they are sometimes referred to as 'neck breathers'. He breathes through a tracheal stoma (hole in front of neck). In these patients give oxygen and, if required, assist ventilation via the stoma, and not the mouth. This can be done by mouth-to-stoma, by holding a small face mask over the stoma, or by inserting a tracheal tube into the stoma, depending on your skills.

Summary learning

- **Airway management and ventilation are essential parts of cardiopulmonary resuscitation.**
- **Airway obstruction can usually be relieved with simple techniques.**
- **Simple adjuncts make airway management more effective and acceptable.**
- **When the skill for tracheal intubation is not available a supraglottic airway is an acceptable alternative.**

My key take-home messages from this chapter

Further reading

Soar J, Callaway CW, Aibiki M, et al. Part 4: Advanced life support: 2015 International Consensus on Cardiopulmonary Resuscitation and Emergency Cardiovascular Care Science With Treatment Recommendations. Resuscitation 2015;95:e71-e122.

Soar J, Nolan JP, Bottiger BW, et al. European Resuscitation Council Guidelines for Resuscitation 2015 Section 3 Adult Advanced Life Support. Resuscitation 2015;95:99-146.

Soar J, Nolan JP. Airway management in cardiopulmonary resuscitation. Curr Opin Crit Care 2013;19:181-7.

Cardiac arrest rhythms – monitoring and recognition

Contents

- **ECG monitoring**
- **Diagnosis from cardiac monitors**
- **Cardiac arrest rhythms**

Learning outcomes

To enable you to:
- **Understand the reasons for ECG monitoring**
- **Monitor the ECG**
- **Recognise the rhythms associated with cardiac arrest**

Introduction

ECG monitoring enables identification of the cardiac rhythm in patients in cardiac arrest. Monitoring patients at risk of developing arrhythmias can enable treatment before cardiac arrest occurs. Patients at risk of cardiac arrest include those with chest pain, collapse or syncope, palpitations, or shock (e.g. due to bleeding or sepsis). Simple, single-lead ECG monitoring will not detect cardiac ischaemia reliably. Record serial 12-lead ECGs in patients experiencing chest pain suggestive of an acute coronary syndrome. In all patients who have persistent arrhythmia (abnormal heart rhythm) and are at risk of deterioration, establish ECG monitoring and as soon as possible record a good-quality 12-lead ECG. Monitoring alone will not always enable accurate rhythm recognition and it is important to document the arrhythmia in 12 leads for future reference if required.

Accurate analysis of cardiac rhythm abnormalities requires experience, but by applying basic principles most rhythms can be interpreted sufficiently to enable selection of the appropriate treatment. The inability to recognise reliably ventricular fibrillation (VF) or other rhythms likely to respond to a shock is a major drawback in the use of manual defibrillators. Automated external defibrillators (AEDs) overcome this problem by automatic analysis of the rhythm. For a shockable rhythm, the defibrillator charges to a pre-determined energy and instructs the operator that a shock is required. The introduction of AEDs has meant that more people can now apply defibrillation safely. People who lack training or confidence in recognising cardiac rhythms should use AEDs.

It may be difficult to diagnose accurately an abnormal peri-arrest rhythm. Nevertheless, by following simple rules, any arrhythmia can be classified sufficiently accurately to enable recognition that the rhythm is abnormal, to assess the effect of the rhythm on the patient's clinical condition, and thus to select appropriate and effective treatment. For example, a precise ECG classification of a bradycardia is usually less important than recognising that the heart rate is inappropriately slow for the patient and starting appropriate treatment with atropine or cardiac pacing. It is equally important to assess the haemodynamic effects of a tachycardia. In many cases the precise treatment for a tachycardia, and the urgency for it, depends greatly on the effects of the arrhythmia on cardiac output. In turn, these depend on the patient's underlying cardiac function; the

ILS

same arrhythmia may have different consequences in different patients. Precise ECG classification of the tachycardia is often less important.

Remember – treat the patient not the ECG

ECG monitoring

Planned ECG monitoring

When there is time to plan ECG monitoring, attach self-adhesive ECG electrodes to the patient's chest. The positions described will allow records that approximate to standard lead I, II, and III of the conventional ECG. Select the configuration that displays the most prominent P waves (if organised atrial activity is present) with sufficient QRS amplitude. This is usually lead II.

The ECG cables are usually colour coded. The red electrode goes to the right shoulder (**Red** to the **Right**), the yellow electrode to the left shoulder (ye**LL**ow to **L**eft), and the green or leg electrode below the pectoral muscles or on the upper abdominal wall (**Green** for le**G**) (Figure 6.1).

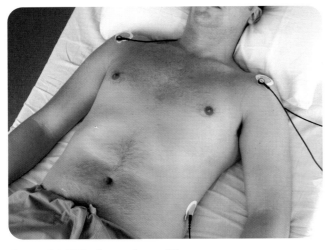

Figure 6.1 ECG electrode positions

Placing the electrodes over bone rather than muscle reduces electrical interference. Leave the precordium unobstructed for chest compression and defibrillation. If possible, shave the areas where the electrodes are attached, and clean the skin with alcohol to dissolve skin oil. Most adhesive electrodes include an electrolyte gel to ensure good electrical contact. Some electrodes have a rough surface on the wrapping, which can be used to gently abrade the skin before the electrode is attached, improving contact. In co-operative patients, reduce movement artefact by keeping them warm and reassured.

Emergency monitoring

In an emergency, such as a collapsed patient, assess the cardiac rhythm as soon as possible by applying self-adhesive defibrillator pads, which can be used for monitoring and hands-free shock delivery (Figure 6.2). The electrodes are applied beneath the right clavicle and the

other over the left lower chest in the mid-axillary line. Monitor the cardiac rhythm continuously with proper ECG electrodes as soon as possible after cardiac arrest.

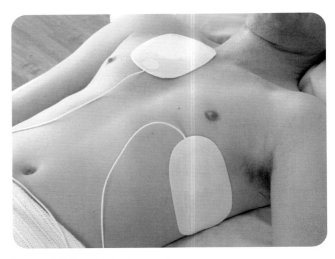

Figure 6.2 Defibrillation pads

Diagnosis from cardiac monitors

The displays and printouts from cardiac monitors are suitable only for recognition of rhythms and not for more detailed ECG interpretation.

Basic electrocardiography

The normal adult heart rate is defined as 60–100 min^{-1}. A rate below 60 min^{-1} is a bradycardia and a rate of 100 min^{-1} or more is a tachycardia. Under normal circumstances depolarisation is initiated from a group of specialised pacemaker cells, the sinoatrial (SA) node, in the right atrium (Figure 6.3). The wave of depolarisation spreads from the SA node into the atrial muscle; this is seen on the ECG as the P wave (Figure 6.4). Atrial contraction is the mechanical response to this electrical impulse.

Spread to the ventricular muscle is along specialised conducting tissue the atrioventricular (AV) node and His-Purkinje system. The bundle of His bifurcates to enable depolarisation to spread into the ventricular muscle along two specialised bundles of conducting tissue the right bundle branch to the right ventricle and the left bundle to the left ventricle.

Depolarisation of the ventricles is reflected in the QRS complex of the ECG. The normal sequence of cardiac depolarisation described above is known as sinus rhythm. The T wave that follows the QRS complex represents ventricular repolarisation.

The specialised cells of the conducting tissue (the AV node and His-Purkinje system) enable coordinated ventricular depolarisation, which is more rapid than uncoordinated depolarisation. With normal depolarisation, the QRS complex is narrow, which is defined as less than 0.12 seconds. If one of the bundle branches is diseased, conduction delay causes a broad QRS complex (i.e. greater than 0.12 seconds (3 small squares on the ECG)).

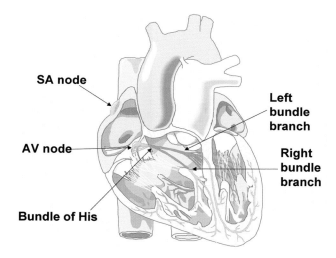

Figure 6.3 Electrical conduction in the heart

SA node

AV node

Bundle of His

Left bundle branch

Right bundle branch

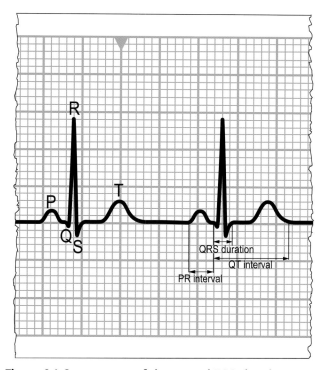

Figure 6.4 Components of the normal ECG signal

Cardiac arrest rhythms

The rhythms present during cardiac arrest are classified into three groups:

- ventricular fibrillation (VF) and pulseless ventricular tachycardia (pVT)

- asystole

- pulseless electrical activity (PEA).

Larger ECG rhythm strips are included at the end of this chapter.

Ventricular fibrillation (VF)

In VF the ventricular myocardium depolarises randomly. The ECG shows rapid, bizarre, irregular waves of widely varying frequency and amplitude (Figure 6.5). VF is sometimes classified as coarse or fine depending on the amplitude (height) of the complexes. If the rhythm is clearly VF (irrespective of coarse or fine), attempt defibrillation.

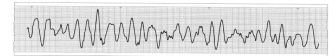

Figure 6.5 Ventricular fibrillation (VF)

Pulseless ventricular tachycardia (pVT)

Ventricular tachycardia, particularly at higher rates or when the left ventricle is compromised, may cause profound loss of cardiac output. Pulseless VT is managed in the same way as VF. The ECG shows a broad-complex tachycardia. In monomorphic VT, the rhythm is regular (or almost regular) at a rate of 100-300 min^{-1} (Figure 6.6).

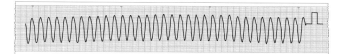

Figure 6.6 Ventricular tachycardia (VT)

Asystole

Usually there is neither atrial nor ventricular activity, and the ECG is a more or less straight line (Figure 6.7). Deflections that can be confused with very fine VF can be caused by baseline drift, electrical interference, respiratory movements, or cardiopulmonary resuscitation. A completely straight line usually means that a monitoring lead has disconnected. Whenever asystole is suspected, check that the gain on the monitor is set correctly (1 mV cm^{-1}) and that the leads are connected correctly. If the monitor has the facility, view another lead configuration.

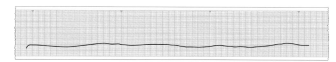

Figure 6.7 Asystole

Atrial activity (i.e. P waves), may continue for a short time after the onset of ventricular asystole: there will be P waves on the ECG but no evidence of ventricular depolarisation (Figure 6.8). These patients may be suitable for cardiac pacing.

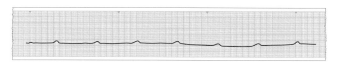

Figure 6.8 Ventricular standstill with continuing sinus P waves

Pulseless electrical activity (PEA)

The term pulseless electrical activity means normal (or near normal) electrical activity without effective cardiac output, and is treated as cardiac arrest. The diagnosis is made when cardiac arrest occurs with a rhythm that would normally be accompanied by a good cardiac output.

Bradycardia

The treatment of bradycardia (a slow heart rate – less than 60 min^{-1}) (Figure 6.9) depends on its haemodynamic consequences. Very slow rates can cause the blood pressure to fall. It is not a true cardiac arrest rhythm as patients usually have a pulse. Bradycardia may however mean imminent cardiac arrest and needs to be treated with atropine or other measures (e.g. pacing) in patients with adverse features (e.g. low blood pressure, fainting, chest pain, heart failure).

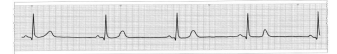

Figure 6.9 Sinus bradycardia

Agonal rhythm

Agonal rhythm is characterised by slow, irregular, wide ventricular complexes of varying shape (Figure 6.10). This does not generate a pulse. It is usually seen during the late stages of unsuccessful resuscitation. The complexes slow inexorably becoming progressively broader until all recognisable electrical activity is lost.

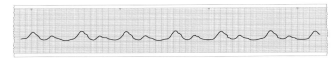

Figure 6.10 Agonal rhythm

Summary learning

- **Monitor the ECG in all patients in cardiac arrest.**
- **Automated external defibrillators (AEDs) will recognise shockable rhythms (VF/pVT) and advise a shock.**

My key take-home messages from this chapter

Rhythm strips

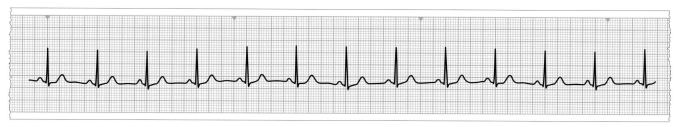

Rhythm strip 1 Sinus rhythm

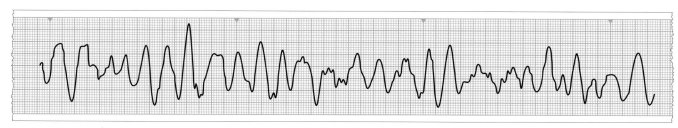

Rhythm strip 2 Coarse ventricular fibrillation

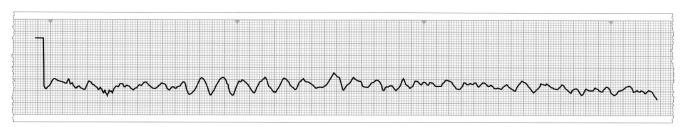

Rhythm strip 3 Fine ventricular fibrillation

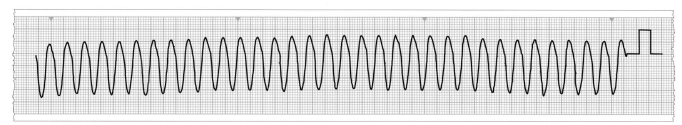

Rhythm strip 4 Ventricular tachycardia

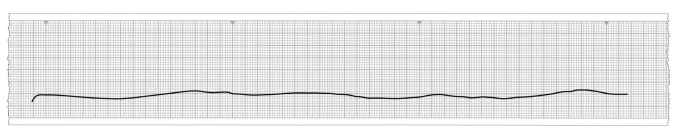

Rhythm strip 5 Asystole

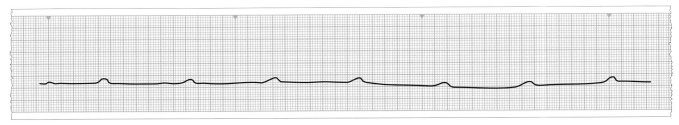

Rhythm strip 6 Ventricular standstill with continuing sinus P waves

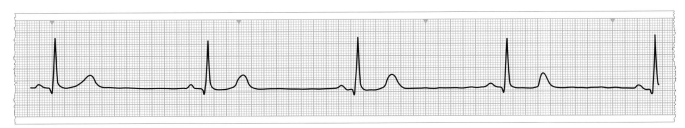

Rhythm strip 7 Sinus bradycardia

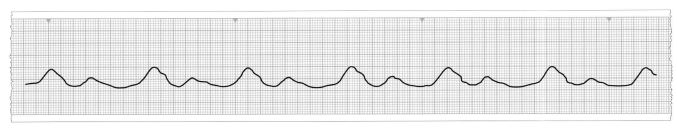

Rhythm strip 8 Agonal rhythm

Defibrillation

Contents

- **The mechanism of defibrillation**
- **Factors affecting the success of defibrillation**
- **Safety during defibrillation**
- **Automated external defibrillators (AEDs) and sequence for use**
- **Manual defibrillation and sequence for use**

Learning outcomes

To enable you to:

- **Understand how to safely deliver a shock with an AED or manual defibrillator**
- **Understand how to minimise pauses in chest compressions during defibrillation**

Introduction

Following the onset of ventricular fibrillation or pulseless ventricular tachycardia (VF/pVT), cardiac output ceases and cerebral hypoxic injury starts within 3 minutes. For complete neurological recovery, early successful defibrillation with return of spontaneous circulation (ROSC) is essential. The shorter the interval between the onset of VF/pVT and delivery of the shock, the greater the chance of successful defibrillation and survival. Defibrillation is a key link in the Chain of Survival and is one of the few interventions proven to improve outcome from VF/pVT cardiac arrest.

For all cardiac arrests:

Start CPR – as soon as a defibrillator arrives attach the defibrillator pads, assess the rhythm and give a shock if indicated.

A manual defibrillator enables you to decide when and how to give the shock.

If you, or your colleagues are not confident in rhythm recognition, use an automated external defibrillator (AED) or a manual defibrillator with an AED mode. Switch the AED on and follow the audiovisual prompts.

Some defibrillators also provide prompts and feedback on the quality of chest compressions. You need to be familiar with the defibrillators you are likely to use in a cardiac arrest.

Mechanism of defibrillation

Defibrillation is the passage of an electrical current across the myocardium to depolarise a critical mass of heart muscle simultaneously, enabling the natural 'pacemaker' tissue to resume control. To achieve this, all defibrillators have:

- a power source capable of providing direct current

- a capacitor that can be charged to a pre-determined energy level

ILS

- two electrodes which are placed on the patient's chest, either side of the heart, across which the capacitor is discharged.

Successful defibrillation is defined as the absence of VF/pVT at 5 seconds after shock delivery, although the ultimate goal is ROSC.

Factors affecting defibrillation success

Defibrillation success depends on sufficient current being delivered to the myocardium. Factors affecting defibrillation success include the transthoracic impedance, electrode position, the shock energy, and the shock sequence.

Transthoracic impedance

Some defibrillators measure the transthoracic impedance and adjust their output accordingly, which is known as impedance compensation. To minimise the impedance:

- Ensure good contact between self-adhesive pads and the patient's skin. Use the self-adhesive pads recommended by the manufacturer for the specific defibrillator.

- If the patient has a very hairy chest and a razor is available immediately, use it to shave the area where the electrodes are placed. Make sure chest compressions continue whilst shaving the chest. However, defibrillation should not be delayed if a razor is not to hand immediately.

- Remove drug patches if in the area where self-adhesive pads would be applied. If this is likely to delay defibrillation, place the pads in an alternative position that avoids the patch.

Electrode position

The electrodes (also called defibrillator pads, self-adhesive pads) are positioned for greatest current flow through the myocardium. The standard positions are one electrode to the right of the upper sternum below the clavicle, and the other (apical) in the mid-axillary line, approximately level with the V6 ECG electrode and clear of breast tissue. The apical electrode must be sufficiently lateral (Figure 7.1). Other acceptable positions include:

- One electrode anteriorly, over the left precordium, and the other electrode on the back behind the heart, just inferior to the left scapula (antero-posterior).

- One electrode placed in the standard apical position, and the other electrode on the back, over the right scapula (postero-lateral).

- The lateral chest walls, one on the right and the other on the left side (bi-axillary).

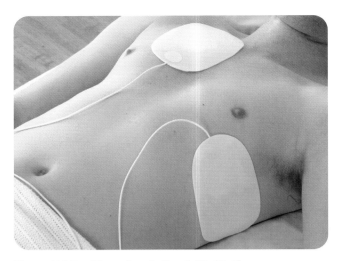

Figure 7.1 Position of pads for defibrillation

If the patient has a pacemaker or similar device, place the pads away from the device (at least 10–15 cm) or use an alternative electrode position (see below).

Shock energy

If you are using an AED, you do not need to choose the shock energy as the AED will do this for you. All you have to do is follow the AED prompts.

If you are using a manual defibrillator you will need to choose the shock energy – give a first shock of at least 150 J. The recommended shock energy varies according to the defibrillator's manufacturer. On some defibrillators the recommended shock energy is readily apparent (e.g. marked on the display or preset). You should be familiar with the defibrillators where you work. If you are unaware of the effective energy dose, use the highest energy setting for the first and subsequent shocks.

If the first shock is unsuccessful, second and subsequent shocks can be delivered using either fixed or increasing energies, depending on the device in use. If a higher energy setting is available it is reasonable to increase the shock energy. If a shockable rhythm recurs (refibrillation) after successful defibrillation (with or without ROSC), give the next shock with a higher energy level if this is feasible.

Shock sequence

For all cardiac arrests start CPR and use the defibrillator to assess the rhythm as soon as it arrives. Although defibrillation is key to the management of patients in VF/pVT, continuous, uninterrupted chest compressions are also required to optimise the chances of successful resuscitation. Even short interruptions in chest compressions (e.g. to deliver rescue breaths or perform rhythm analysis) reduce the chances of successful defibrillation. The aim is to ensure that chest compressions are performed continuously throughout the resuscitation attempt, pausing briefly only to enable specific interventions.

Another factor that is critical in determining the success of defibrillation is the duration of the interval between stopping chest compressions and delivering the shock: the pre-shock pause. Every 5-second increase in the pre-shock pause almost halves the chance of successful defibrillation. Consequently, defibrillation must always be performed quickly and efficiently in order to maximise the chances of successful resuscitation. If there is any delay in obtaining a defibrillator, and while the defibrillator pads are being applied, start chest compressions and ventilation.

The precise sequence for giving shocks with an AED and manual defibrillator is described below.

Safety

Do not deliver a shock if anybody is touching the patient. Do not hold intravenous infusion equipment or the patient's trolley during shock delivery. The operator must ensure that everyone is clear of the patient before delivering a shock. Wipe any water or fluids from the patient's chest before attempted defibrillation. The gloves routinely available in clinical settings do not provide sufficient protection from the electric current, therefore a shock is delivered only when everyone is clear of the patient.

Safe use of oxygen during defibrillation

Sparks in an oxygen-enriched atmosphere can cause fire and burns to the patient. Self-adhesive pads are far less likely to cause sparks than manual paddles – no fires have been reported in association with the use of self-adhesive pads. The following precautions reduce the risk of fire:

- Remove any oxygen mask or nasal cannulae and place them at least 1 metre away from the patient's chest.

- Leave the self-inflating bag connected to the tracheal tube or supraglottic airway. No increase in oxygen concentration occurs in the zone of defibrillation, even with an oxygen flow of 15 L min^{-1}. Alternatively, disconnect the ventilation bag from the tracheal tube or supraglottic airway and remove it at least 1 metre from the patient's chest during defibrillation.

- If the patient is connected to a ventilator, for example in the operating room or critical care unit, leave the ventilator tubing (breathing circuit) connected to the tracheal tube unless chest compressions prevent the ventilator from delivering adequate tidal volumes. In this case, the ventilator is usually substituted by a self-inflating bag, which can be left connected or detached and removed to a distance of at least 1 metre. If the ventilator tubing is disconnected, ensure that it is kept at least 1 metre from the patient or, better still, switch the ventilator off; modern ventilators generate massive oxygen flows when disconnected.

Automated external defibrillators

Automated external defibrillators are sophisticated, reliable, computerised devices that use voice and visual prompts to guide lay rescuers and healthcare professionals to attempt defibrillation safely in cardiac arrest victims (Figure 7.2).

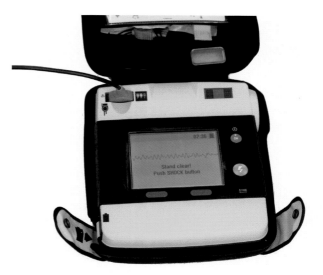

Figure 7.2 Automated external defibrillator (AED)

Automated rhythm analysis

It is almost impossible to shock inappropriately with an AED. Movement is usually sensed, so movement artefact is unlikely to be interpreted as a shockable rhythm.

In-hospital use of AEDs

Delayed defibrillation can occur when cardiac arrest occurs in unmonitored clinical areas or non-clinical areas. Several minutes may elapse before the resuscitation team arrives with a defibrillator and delivers shocks. AEDs enable rapid defibrillation in areas where staff have no rhythm recognition skills. Sufficient staff should be trained to enable the first shock to be delivered within 3 minutes of collapse anywhere in the hospital.

In hospital areas where there is rapid access to manual defibrillation, either from trained staff or a resuscitation team, use manual defibrillation in preference to an AED. Ensure that an effective system for training and retraining is in place. Healthcare providers with a duty to perform CPR should be trained, equipped, and authorised to perform defibrillation, and sufficient numbers should be trained to enable the first shock to be delivered within 3 minutes of collapse anywhere in the hospital.

Public access defibrillation (PAD) programmes

Public access defibrillation (PAD) and first responder AED programmes may increase the number of victims who receive bystander CPR and early defibrillation, thus improving survival from out-of-hospital cardiac arrest. These programmes require an organised and practised response with rescuers trained and equipped to recognise emergencies, activate the emergency medical services (EMS) system, provide CPR, and use the AED. Lay rescuer

AED programmes with very rapid response times in locations (e.g. in airports, railway stations, bus terminals, sport facilities, shopping malls, casinos) where cardiac arrests are usually witnessed and trained CPR providers can quickly be on scene report high survival rates for VF/pVT cardiac arrest. Registration of AEDs for public access, so that dispatchers can direct bystanders to a nearby AED, may also help to optimise response.

More recently, there has been greater emphasis on training lay people to learn CPR and encourage people to use AEDs available in public places, even if they have had no previous training. This is because even untrained individuals who switch on an AED and follow the prompts can save the life of a person in cardiac arrest.

Sequence for use of an AED

It is critically important that CPR providers pay attention to AED voice prompts and follow them without any delay.

1. Make sure the victim, any bystanders, and you are safe.

2. If the victim is unresponsive and not breathing normally:

   - ask someone to call for an ambulance or the resuscitation team and collect the AED. If you are on your own, do this yourself.

3. Start CPR according to the guidelines (Chapter 3).

4. As soon as the AED arrives:

   - switch on the AED and attach the electrode pads.

   - if more than one rescuer is present, continue CPR while this is done (Figure 7.3 a).

   - follow the voice/visual directions.

   - ensure that nobody touches the victim whilst the AED is analysing the rhythm (Figure 7.3 b).

5A. If a shock IS indicated:

   - ensure that nobody touches the victim.

   - push the shock button as directed (Figure 7.3 c).

   - continue as directed by the voice/visual prompts.

5B. If NO shock is indicated:

   - immediately resume CPR using a ratio of 30 compressions to 2 rescue breaths (Figure 7.3 d).

   - continue as directed by the voice/visual prompts.

6. Continue to follow the AED prompts until:

   - qualified help (e.g. ambulance or resuscitation team) arrives and takes over,

   - the victim starts to breathe normally, or

   - you become exhausted.

- The carrying case with the AED must contain strong scissors for cutting through clothing and a disposable razor for shaving excessive chest hair in order to obtain good electrode contact.

- If ALS providers are using an AED, they should use other ALS interventions (e.g. advanced airway techniques, ventilation, IV access, drug delivery, etc.) according to local protocols.

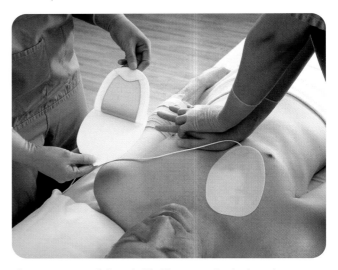

Figure 7.3a Applying defibrillator pads during chest compressions

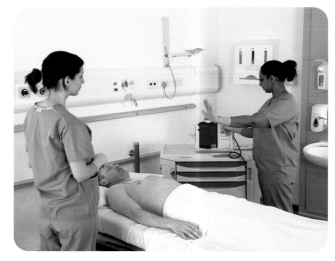

Figure 7.3b Everyone clear while the AED analyses the rhythm

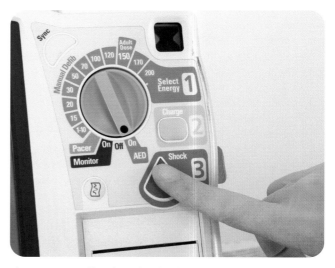

Figure 7.3c Delivering shock when prompted by AED

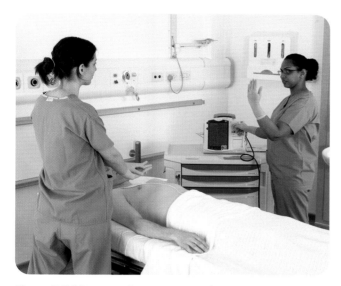

Figure 7.3d Restart chest compressions

Manual defibrillation

Manual defibrillators have some advantages over AEDs. They enable the operator to diagnose the rhythm and deliver a shock rapidly without having to wait for rhythm analysis. This minimises the interruption in chest compressions. Manual defibrillators often have additional functions, such as the ability to deliver synchronised shocks, and external pacing. The main disadvantage is that the operator has to be skilled in ECG rhythm recognition.

Sequence for use of a manual defibrillator

This sequence is an integral part of the Advanced Life Support treatment algorithm in Chapter 4.

1. Confirm cardiac arrest – check for signs of life or if trained to do so, normal breathing and pulse simultaneously.

2. Call the resuscitation team.

3. Perform uninterrupted chest compressions while applying self-adhesive defibrillation/monitoring pads (Figure 7.4a) – one below the right clavicle and the other in the V6 position in the midaxillary line.

4. Plan actions before pausing CPR for rhythm analysis and communicate these to the team.

5. Stop chest compressions; confirm VF/pVT from the ECG. Ensure that this pause in chest compressions is brief and no longer than 5 seconds.

6. Resume chest compressions immediately; warn all rescuers **other than the individual performing the chest compressions** to "stand clear" (Figure 7.4b) and remove any oxygen delivery device as appropriate.

7. The designated person selects the appropriate energy on the defibrillator and presses the charge button. Choose an energy setting of at least 150 J for the first shock, the same or a higher energy for subsequent shocks, or follow the manufacturer's guidance for the particular defibrillator.

8. Ensure that the rescuer giving the compressions is the only person touching the patient.

9. Once the defibrillator is charged and the safety check is complete, tell the rescuer doing the chest compressions to "stand clear" (Figure 7.4c); when clear, give the shock.

10. After shock delivery immediately restart CPR using a ratio of 30:2, starting with chest compressions (Figure 7.4d). Do not pause to reassess the rhythm or feel for a pulse. This pause in chest compressions should be brief and no longer than 5 seconds.

11. Continue CPR for 2 minutes; the team leader prepares the team for the next pause in CPR.

12. Pause briefly to check the monitor.

13. If VF/pVT, repeat steps 6–12 above and deliver a second shock.

14. If VF/pVT persists repeat steps 6–8 above and deliver a third shock. Resume chest compressions immediately. Give adrenaline 1 mg IV and amiodarone 300 mg IV while performing a further 2 minutes CPR. Withhold adrenaline if there are signs of ROSC during CPR.

15. Repeat this 2 minutes CPR – rhythm/pulse check – defibrillation sequence if VF/pVT persists.

16. Give further adrenaline 1 mg IV after alternate shocks (i.e. approximately every 3–5 minutes).

17. If organised electrical activity compatible with a cardiac output is seen during a rhythm check, seek evidence of ROSC (check for signs of life, a central pulse and end-tidal CO_2 if available).

    – If there is ROSC, start post-resuscitation care.

    – If there are no signs of ROSC, continue CPR and switch to the non-shockable algorithm.

18. If asystole is seen, continue CPR and switch to the non-shockable algorithm.

Witnessed and monitored VF/pVT cardiac arrest

If a patient has a monitored and witnessed cardiac arrest in the catheter laboratory, coronary care unit, a critical care area, or whilst monitored after cardiac surgery, and a manual defibrillator is rapidly available:

- Confirm cardiac arrest and shout for help.

- If the initial rhythm is VF/pVT, give up to three quick successive (stacked) shocks.

- Rapidly check for a rhythm change and, if appropriate check for a pulse and other signs of ROSC after each defibrillation attempt.

- Start chest compressions and continue CPR for 2 minutes if the third shock is unsuccessful.

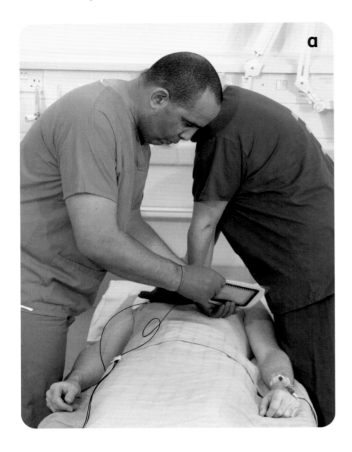

This three-shock strategy may also be considered for an initial, witnessed VF/pVT cardiac arrest if the patient is already connected to a manual defibrillator – these circumstances are rare. There are no data supporting a three-shock strategy in any of these circumstances, but it is unlikely that chest compressions will improve the already very high chance of ROSC when defibrillation occurs early, immediately after onset of VF/pVT.

Synchronised cardioversion

For patients not in cardiac arrest, a manual defibrillator can be used for synchronised cardioversion. If electrical cardioversion is used to convert atrial or ventricular tachyarrhythmias, the shock must be synchronised with the R wave (not the T wave) of the ECG. By avoiding the relative refractory period, the risk of inducing VF is minimised. Most manual defibrillators have a switch that enables the shock to be triggered by the R wave on the ECG. Electrodes are applied to the chest wall and cardioversion is achieved in the same way as attempted defibrillation, but the operator must anticipate the slight delay between pressing the buttons and the discharge of the shock when the next R wave occurs.

With some defibrillators, the synchronised mode has to be reset if a second shock is required. Other machines remain in the synchronised mode; be careful not to leave the synchronisation switch in the 'on' position following use as this will inhibit discharge of the defibrillator when it is next used for treating VF/pVT.

Implanted electronic devices

When a patient needs external defibrillation, effective measures to try to restore life take priority over concerns about any implanted device such as a pacemaker, implantable cardioverter-defibrillator (ICD), implantable event recorder or neurostimulator. Current resuscitation guidelines are followed, but awareness of the presence of an implanted device allows some additional measures to optimise outcome:

- To minimise the risk of damage to the device, place the defibrillator electrodes away from the pacemaker or ICD generator (at least 10–15 cm) without compromising

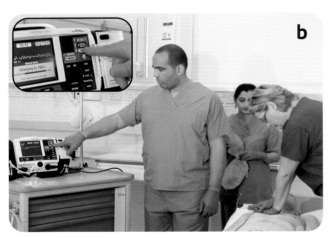

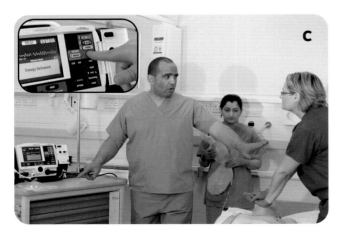

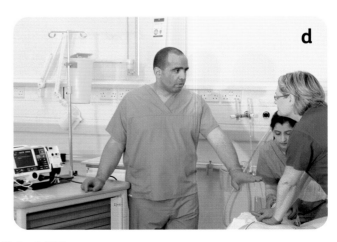

Figures 7.4 a, b, c, d Operation of a manual defibrillator and efficient CPR

effective defibrillation. If necessary place the pads in the antero-posterior, postero-lateral or bi-axillary position as described above.

- An ICD gives no warning when it delivers a shock. In an emergency, a ring magnet can be placed over the ICD to disable the defibrillation function if required. Deactivation of an ICD in this way does not disable the ability of the device to act as a pacemaker if it has that capability.

- During in a shockable rhythm, external defibrillation should be attempted in the usual way if the ICD has not delivered a shock, or if its shocks have failed to terminate the arrhythmia.

Summary learning

- **For the patient in VF, early defibrillation is the only effective means of restoring a spontaneous circulation.**

- **When using a defibrillator, minimise interruptions in chest compressions.**

- **Use an AED if you are not confident in rhythm recognition or manual defibrillation.**

My key take-home messages from this chapter

Further reading

Cardiovascular implanted electronic devices in people towards the end of life, during cardiopulmonary resuscitation and after death. Guidance from the Resuscitation Council (UK), British Cardiovascular Society and National Council for Palliative Care. March 2015.
https://www.resus.org.uk/defibrillators/cardiovascular-implanted-electronic-devices/

Soar J, Callaway CW, Aibiki M, et al. Part 4: Advanced life support: 2015 International Consensus on Cardiopulmonary Resuscitation and Emergency Cardiovascular Care Science With Treatment Recommendations. Resuscitation 2015;95:e71-e122.

Soar J, Nolan JP, Bottiger BW, et al. European Resuscitation Council Guidelines for Resuscitation 2015 Section 3 Adult Advanced Life Support. Resuscitation 2015;95:99-146.

Post-resuscitation care

Contents

- **The post-cardiac arrest syndrome**
- **The post-resuscitation care algorithm**
- **Optimising organ function**
- **Prognostication**

Learning outcomes

To enable you to:

- **Understand the need for continued resuscitation after return of spontaneous circulation**
- **Understand the post-cardiac arrest syndrome**
- **Facilitate transfer of the patient safely**
- **Consider the role and limitations of assessing prognosis after cardiac arrest**

Introduction

Immediate Life Support (ILS) skills may be successful before expert help arrives. Return of a spontaneous circulation (ROSC) is an important first step, but the ultimate goal of resuscitation is to return the patient to a state of normal cerebral function, and to establish and maintain a stable cardiac rhythm and normal haemodynamic function. The post-resuscitation care algorithm (Figure 8.1) shows the key steps for a successful outcome. Many of the interventions are complex and require specialist help and are provided here as an overview to the topic. As an ILS provider you would only need to know the immediate steps. Make sure you have called for help so the patient gets the appropriate treatments. Many of the interventions (e.g. interventional cardiology, intensive care, neurophysiology) are available only in specialist centres and it is likely that over time patients who have an out-of-hospital cardiac arrest will be taken to regional specialist Cardiac Arrest Centres.

The quality of treatment provided in this post-resuscitation phase – the final ring in the Chain of Survival – significantly influences the patient's ultimate outcome. The post-resuscitation phase starts at the location where ROSC is achieved but, once stabilised, transfer the patient to the most appropriate high-care area (e.g. intensive care unit (ICU), coronary care unit (CCU)) for further treatment.

You will need expert help for the post-resuscitation care of survivors from cardiac arrest.

The post-cardiac arrest syndrome

The post-cardiac arrest syndrome comprises:

- post-cardiac arrest brain injury
- post-cardiac arrest myocardial dysfunction

ILS

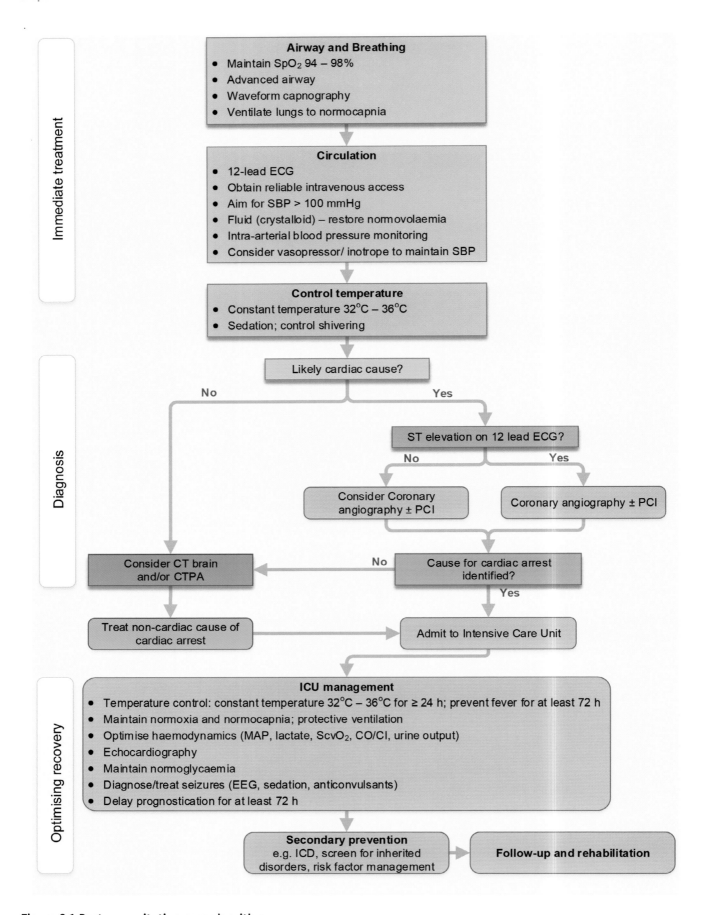

Figure 8.1 Post-resuscitation care algorithm
SBP systolic blood pressure; **PCI** percutaneous coronary intervention; **CTPA** computed tomography pulmonary angiogram;
ICU Intensive care unit; **MAP** mean arterial pressure; **ScvO₂** central venous oxygenation; **CO/CI** cardiac output/cardiac index;
EEG electroencephalography; **ICD** implanted cardioverter defibrillator.

- systemic ischaemia/reperfusion response
- persistent precipitating pathology.

The severity of this syndrome will vary with the duration and cause of cardiac arrest. It may not occur at all if the cardiac arrest is brief:

- Post-cardiac arrest brain injury manifests as coma, seizures, myoclonus, varying degrees of neurological dysfunction and brain death.

- Significant myocardial dysfunction is common after cardiac arrest but typically recovers by 2-3 days.

- The whole body ischaemia/reperfusion that occurs with resuscitation from cardiac arrest activates immunological and coagulation pathways contributing to multiple organ failure and increasing the risk of infection.

- The persistent precipitating pathology is what caused the cardiac arrest in the first place. For example if the patient had a myocardial infarction this would have an impact on the heart function.

- The post-cardiac arrest syndrome has many features in common with sepsis, including intravascular volume depletion and vasodilation.

Continued resuscitation

In the immediate post-resuscitation phase treat the patient by following the ABCDE approach (Figure 8.2).

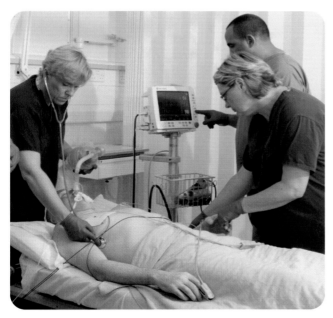

Figure 8.2 The ABCDE approach to post-resuscitation care

Airway and breathing
Aim: to ensure a clear airway, adequate oxygenation and ventilation.

Patients who have had a brief period of cardiac arrest that responded immediately to appropriate treatment (e.g.

witnessed ventricular fibrillation (VF) reverting to sinus rhythm after early defibrillation) may achieve an immediate return of normal cerebral function. These patients do not require tracheal intubation and ventilation, but should be given oxygen by face mask if needed to maintain a normal arterial oxygen saturation. Other patients may not be immediately neurologically normal, even after a rapid successful resuscitation. Hypoxia and hypercarbia both increase the likelihood of a further cardiac arrest and can cause secondary brain injury. Recent studies suggest that high levels of oxygen in the blood (hyperoxaemia) after resuscitation from cardiac arrest can also be harmful.

As soon as arterial blood oxygen saturation can be monitored reliably (by blood gas analysis and/or pulse oximetry (SpO_2)), titrate the inspired oxygen concentration to maintain the arterial blood oxygen saturation in the range of 94–98%. Consider tracheal intubation, sedation and controlled ventilation in patients with obtunded cerebral function. This requires expert help. The patient's lungs are ventilated aiming to achieve a normal arterial blood carbon dioxide concentration ($PaCO_2$).

Examine the patient's chest and look for symmetrical chest movement. Listen to ensure that the breath sounds are equal on both sides. A tracheal tube that has been inserted too far will tend to go down the right main bronchus and fail to ventilate the left lung. If ribs have been fractured during chest compression there may be a pneumothorax (reduced or absent breath sounds) or a flail segment. Listen for evidence of pulmonary oedema or pulmonary aspiration of gastric contents. Insert a gastric tube – this will decompress the stomach following mouth-to-mouth or bag-mask ventilation, prevent splinting of the diaphragm, and enable drainage of gastric contents.

If the intubated patient regains consciousness soon after ROSC, is cooperative and breathing normally, consider immediate extubation: coughing on the tracheal tube may provoke arrhythmias and, or hypertension. If immediate or early extubation is not possible, sedate the patient to ensure the tracheal tube is tolerated, and provide ventilatory support.

Circulation
Aim: the maintenance of normal sinus rhythm and a cardiac output adequate for perfusion of vital organs.

Cardiac rhythm and blood pressure are likely to be unstable following a cardiac arrest. Continuous monitoring of the ECG is essential. Record the pulse and blood pressure and assess peripheral perfusion: warm, pink fingers with a rapid capillary refill usually imply adequate perfusion. Grossly distended neck veins when the patient is semi-upright may indicate right ventricular failure, but in rare cases could indicate pericardial tamponade. Left ventricular failure may be indicated by fine inspiratory crackles heard on auscultation of the lungs, and the production of pink frothy sputum. If the facility for direct continuous arterial blood pressure monitoring is available insert an arterial cannula to enable reliable monitoring during transfer. Once in a high-care area, the use of non-invasive cardiac output monitoring devices is useful. Infusion of fluids may be required to increase right heart filling pressures or conversely, diuretics and vasodilators may be needed to treat left ventricular failure.

Record a 12-lead ECG as soon as possible. Acute ST-segment elevation or new left bundle branch block in a patient with a typical history of acute myocardial infarction is an indication for treatment to try to re-open an occluded coronary artery (reperfusion therapy) – this is usually achieved by emergency percutaneous coronary intervention (PCI). Services should aim to achieve a 'call-to-balloon' time (i.e. time from call for help to attempted re-opening of the culprit artery) of < 120 minutes whenever possible. Consider fibrinolytic therapy if this is not possible. Cardiopulmonary resuscitation, even if prolonged, is not a contraindication to fibrinolytic therapy.

In post-resuscitation patients, chest pain and/or ST elevation are relatively poor predictors of acute coronary occlusion; for this reason primary PCI should be considered in all post-resuscitation patients who are suspected of having coronary artery disease as the cause of their arrest, even if they are sedated and mechanically ventilated. Several studies indicate that the combination of therapeutic hypothermia (see below) and PCI is feasible and safe after cardiac arrest caused by acute myocardial infarction.

Disability and exposure

Aim: to evaluate the neurological function and ensure that cardiac arrest has not been associated with other medical or surgical conditions requiring immediate treatment.

Although cardiac arrest is caused frequently by primary cardiac disease, other precipitating conditions must be excluded, particularly in hospital patients (e.g. massive blood loss, respiratory failure, pulmonary embolism). Assess the other body systems rapidly so that further resuscitation is appropriate for the patient's needs. To examine the patient properly full exposure of the body may be necessary.

Although it may not be of immediate significance to the patient's management, assess neurological function rapidly and record the Glasgow Coma Scale score (GCS) (Table 8.1). The maximum score possible is 15; the minimum score possible is 3.

Consider the need for targeted temperature management (TTM) in any patient who remains comatose after initial resuscitation from cardiac arrest (see below). When TTM is considered an appropriate treatment, start it as soon as possible – do not wait until the patient is in the ICU before starting to cool a patient.

Glasgow Coma Scale score		
Eye opening	Spontaneously	4
	To speech	3
	To pain	2
	Nil	1
Verbal	Orientated	5
	Confused	4
	Inappropriate words	3
	Incomprehensible sounds	2
	Nil	1
Best motor response	Obeys commands	6
	Localises	5
	Normal flexion	4
	Abnormal flexion	3
	Extension	2
	Nil	1

Table 8.1 The Glasgow Coma Scale score

Further assessment

History
Aim: To establish the patient's state of health and regular drug therapy before the cardiac arrest.

Obtain a comprehensive history as quickly as possible. Those involved in caring for the patient immediately before the cardiac arrest may be able to help (e.g. paramedics, ward staff, and relatives). Ask specifically about symptoms of cardiac disease. If primary cardiac disease seems unlikely, consider other causes of cardiac arrest (e.g. drug overdose, subarachnoid haemorrhage). Make a note of any delay before the start of resuscitation, and the duration of the resuscitation; this may have prognostic significance, although is generally unreliable and certainly should not be used alone to predict outcome. The patient's baseline physiological reserve (before the cardiac arrest) is one of the most important factors taken into consideration by the ICU team when determining whether prolonged multiple organ support is appropriate.

Monitoring
Aim: to enable continuous assessment of vital organ function and to identify trends.

Continuous monitoring of ECG, arterial and possibly central venous blood pressures, respiratory rate, pulse oximetry, capnography, core temperature and urinary output is essential to detect changes during the period of instability that follows resuscitation from cardiac arrest. Monitor continuously the effects of medical interventions (e.g. assisted ventilation, diuretic therapy). This will require expert help.

Investigations

Several physiological variables may be abnormal immediately after a cardiac arrest and urgent biochemical and cardiological investigations should be undertaken (Table 8.2).

Investigations after restoration of circulation	
Full blood count	To exclude anaemia as contributor to myocardial ischaemia and provide baseline values
Biochemistry	To assess renal function To assess electrolyte concentrations (K^+, Mg^{2+}, and Ca^{2+}) To ensure normoglycaemia To commence serial cardiac troponin measurements To provide baseline values
12-lead ECG	To record cardiac rhythm To look for evidence of acute coronary syndrome To look for evidence of old myocardial infarction To provide a baseline record
Chest radiograph	To establish the position of a tracheal tube, a gastric tube, and/or a central venous catheter To check for evidence of pulmonary oedema To check for evidence of pulmonary aspiration To exclude pneumothorax To assess cardiac contour (accurate assessment of heart size requires standard PA erect radiograph – not always practicable in the post-resuscitation situation)
Arterial blood gases	To ensure adequacy of ventilation and oxygenation To ensure correction of acid/base imbalance
Echocardiography	To identify contributing causes to cardiac arrest To assess LV and RV structure and function

Table 8.2 Investigations after restoration of circulation

Patient transfer

Aim: to transfer the patient safely between the site of resuscitation and a place of definitive care.

Following the period of initial post-resuscitation care and stabilisation, the patient will need to be transferred to an appropriate critical care setting (e.g. ICU or CCU). The decision to transfer should be made only after discussion with senior members of the admitting team. Handover care using SBAR or RSVP (Chapter 1). Continue all established monitoring during the transfer and secure all cannulae, catheters, tubes and drains. Make a full re-assessment immediately before the patient is transferred. Ensure that portable suction apparatus, an oxygen supply and a defibrillator and monitor accompany the patient and transfer team.

The transfer team should comprise individuals capable of monitoring the patient and responding appropriately to any change in patient condition, including a further cardiac arrest. The Intensive Care Society (UK) has published guidelines for the transport of the critically ill adult (www.ics.ac.uk). These outline the requirements for equipment and personnel when transferring critically ill patients.

Optimising organ function

Aim: to optimise vital organ function and limit secondary organ damage.

The extent of secondary organ injury after ROSC depends on the ability to minimise the harmful consequences of post-cardiac arrest syndrome. There are several ways to limit the insult to organs following cardiac arrest.

Heart and cardiovascular system

Post-resuscitation myocardial dysfunction causes haemodynamic instability, which manifests as hypotension, a low cardiac output and arrhythmias. Early echocardiography will enable the degree of myocardial dysfunction to be quantified. Treatment with fluid, inotropes and vasopressors may be guided by blood pressure, heart rate, urine output, and rate of plasma lactate clearance and central venous oxygen saturations. Fluids, inotropes and vasopressors may be needed.

In the absence of definitive data supporting a specific goal for blood pressure, target the mean arterial blood pressure to achieve an adequate urine output (1 mL kg^{-1} h^{-1}) and normal or decreasing plasma lactate values, taking into consideration the patient's normal blood pressure, the cause of the arrest and the severity of any myocardial dysfunction. These targets may vary depending on individual physiology and co-morbid status but a systolic blood pressure of at least 100 mmHg is usually required.

Referral for implantable cardioverter defibrillator

Consider the need for an implantable cardioverter defibrillator (ICD) in any patient who has been resuscitated from a primary cardiac arrest. Refer before discharge from hospital to a cardiologist with expertise in heart rhythm disorders.

Brain: optimising neurological recovery

Cerebral perfusion

Immediately after ROSC there is a period of cerebral hyperaemia (increased brain blood flow) followed by low blood flow. Normal cerebral autoregulation is lost, leaving cerebral perfusion dependent on mean arterial pressure. Under these circumstances, hypotension will compromise cerebral blood flow severely and will worsen any brain injury. Try to maintain mean arterial pressure at the patient's normal level.

Sedation

Ventilated patients need to be well-sedated during treatment with targeted temperature management, and the duration of sedation and ventilation is therefore influenced by this treatment. Short-acting drugs (e.g. propofol, alfentanil, remifentanil) will enable earlier neurological assessment. Adequate sedation will reduce oxygen consumption. During hypothermia, optimal sedation can reduce or prevent shivering, which enables the target temperature to be achieved more rapidly.

Control of seizures

Seizures or myoclonus or both occur in one-third of adult patients who achieve ROSC and remain comatose. Seizures increase cerebral metabolism by up to three-fold and may cause cerebral injury: treat with sodium valproate, levetiracetam, phenytoin, benzodiazepines, propofol, or a barbiturate. Myoclonus can be particularly difficult to treat; phenytoin is often ineffective. Propofol is effective to suppress post-anoxic myoclonus. Clonazepam, sodium valproate and levetiracetam are antimyoclonic drugs that may be effective in post-anoxic myoclonus.

Glucose control

A high blood glucose after resuscitation from cardiac arrest is associated with a poor neurological outcome. However, severe hypoglycaemia is also associated with increased mortality in critically ill patients. Following ROSC, blood glucose should be maintained at ≤10 mmol L^{-1}. Hypoglycaemia (< 4.0 mmol L^{-1}) must be avoided.

Temperature control

Treatment of hyperpyrexia

Hyperthermia (hyperpyrexia) is common in the first 48 hours after cardiac arrest and associated with a worse outcome. Treat any hyperthermia occurring after cardiac arrest with antipyretics or active cooling.

Targeted temperature management (TTM)

- Maintain a constant, target temperature between 32°C–36°C for those patients in whom temperature control is used.
- TTM is recommended for adults after out-of-hospital cardiac arrest with an initial shockable rhythm who remain unresponsive after ROSC.
- TTM is suggested for adults after out-of-hospital cardiac arrest with an initial non-shockable rhythm who remain unresponsive after ROSC.
- TTM is suggested for adults after in-hospital cardiac arrest with any initial rhythm who remain unresponsive after ROSC.
- If TTM is used, it is suggested that the duration is at least 24 hours.

Following the TTM trial, 36°C is becoming the preferred target temperature for post-cardiac arrest temperature control. This has several advantages compared with a target temperature of 33°C:

- There is a reduced need for vasopressor support.
- Lactate values are lower (the clinical significance of this is unclear).
- The rewarming phase is shorter.
- There is reduced risk or rebound hyperthermia after rewarming.

How to control temperature

A target temperature of 36°C is not the same as normothermia and in most cases will still require cooling and active temperature management to achieve and maintain this target.

The practical application of TTM is divided into three phases: induction, maintenance and rewarming. External and/or internal cooling techniques can be used to initiate and maintain TTM.

Methods of inducing and/or maintaining TTM include:

- IV infusion of cold fluids with close monitoring to prevent fluid overload to lower temperature.
- Simple ice packs and/or wet towels are inexpensive; however, these methods may be more time consuming for nursing staff, may result in greater temperature fluctuations, and do not enable controlled rewarming.
- Cooling blankets or pads.
- Water or air circulating blankets.
- Water circulating gel-coated pads.
- Transnasal evaporative cooling.
- Intravascular heat exchanger, placed usually in the femoral or subclavian veins.
- Extracorporeal circulation (e.g. cardiopulmonary bypass, ECMO).

In most cases, it is easy to cool patients initially after ROSC because the temperature normally decreases within the first hour. If a target temperature of 36°C is chosen allow a slow passive rewarm to 36°C.

Rebound hyperthermia is associated with worse neurological outcome. Thus, rewarming should be achieved slowly: the optimal rate is not known, but the consensus is currently about 0.25-0.5°C of rewarming per hour.

Prognostication

The prognostication of comatose post-cardiac arrest patients is very complex, should only be undertaken by experienced clinicians and is outside the scope of ILS. This brief summary covers only the broad concepts of prognostication.

Two thirds of those dying after admission to ICU following out-of-hospital cardiac arrest die from neurological injury. Most of these deaths are due to active withdrawal of life sustaining treatment (WLST) based on prognostication of a poor neurological outcome. For this reason, when dealing with patients who are comatose after resuscitation from cardiac arrest minimising the risk of a falsely pessimistic prediction is essential. When predicting a poor outcome these tests should have 100% specificity or zero false positive rate (FPR) (i.e. no individual should have treatment stopped and die when they would have actually had a good outcome). None of the available tests can achieve this.

Prognostication of the comatose post-cardiac arrest patient should be multimodal, in other words involve multiple types of tests of brain injury, and should be delayed sufficiently to enable full clearance of sedatives and any neurological recovery to occur – in most cases, prognostication is not reliable until after 72 hours from cardiac arrest. The tests are categorised:

- clinical examination – GCS score, pupillary response to light, corneal reflex, presence of seizures

- neurophysiological studies – somatosensory evoked potentials (SSEPs) and electroencephalography (EEG)

- biochemical markers – neuron-specific enolase (NSE) is the most commonly used

- imaging studies – brain CT and magnetic resonance imaging (MRI).

Rehabilitation

Although neurological outcome is considered to be good for most cardiac arrest survivors, cognitive and emotional problems and fatigue are common. Long-term cognitive impairments are present in half of survivors. Memory is most frequently affected, followed by problems in attention and executive functioning (i.e. planning and organisation). The cognitive impairments can be severe, but are mostly mild. These patients may benefit from a formal program of rehabilitation.

Organ donation

Post-cardiac arrest patients who do not survive represent an opportunity to increase the number of potential organ donors either after brain death or as 'non-heart-beating' donors.

Care of the resuscitation team

- Audit all resuscitation attempts and, ideally, send these data to the National Cardiac Arrest Audit (Chapter 1).

- Whether the resuscitation attempt was successful or not, the patient's relatives will require considerable support. Consider the pastoral needs of all those associated with the arrest.

Summary learning

- After cardiac arrest, return of spontaneous circulation is just the first stage in a continuum of resuscitation.
- The quality of post-resuscitation care will influence significantly the patient's final outcome.
- These patients require appropriate monitoring, safe transfer to a critical care environment, and continued organ support.
- The post-cardiac arrest syndrome comprises post-cardiac arrest brain injury, post-cardiac arrest myocardial dysfunction, the systemic ischaemia/reperfusion response, and persistence of precipitating pathology.
- Prognosticating the final neurological outcome for those patients remaining comatose after cardiopulmonary resuscitation is complex.

My key take-home messages from this chapter

Further reading

Nielsen N, Wetterslev J, Cronberg T, et al. Targeted temperature management at 33 degrees C versus 36 degrees C after cardiac arrest. N Engl J Med 2013;369:2197-206.

Nolan JP, Soar J, Cariou A, et al. European Resuscitation Council and European Society of Intensive Care Medicine Guidelines for Resuscitation 2015 Section 5 Post Resuscitation Care. Resuscitation 2015;95:201-21.

Soar J, Callaway CW, Aibiki M, et al. Part 4: Advanced life support: 2015 International Consensus on Cardiopulmonary Resuscitation and Emergency Cardiovascular Care Science With Treatment Recommendations. Resuscitation 2015;95:e71-e122.

Sandroni C, Cariou A, Cavallaro F, et al. Prognostication in comatose survivors of cardiac arrest: an advisory statement from the European Resuscitation Council and the European Society of Intensive Care Medicine. Resuscitation 2014;85:1779-89.

Nolan JP, Neumar RW, Adrie C, et al. Post-cardiac arrest syndrome: epidemiology, pathophysiology, treatment, and prognostication. A Scientific Statement from the International Liaison Committee on Resuscitation; the American Heart Association Emergency Cardiovascular Care Committee; the Council on Cardiovascular Surgery and Anesthesia; the Council on Cardiopulmonary, Perioperative, and Critical Care; the Council on Clinical Cardiology; the Council on Stroke. Resuscitation 2008;79:350-79.

Pulse oximetry and oxygen therapy

Contents

- **Pulse oximetry**
- **Targeted oxygen therapy**

Learning outcomes

To enable you to:

- **Understand the principles of pulse oximetry**
- **Understand how to use oxygen safely and effectively**

Role of pulse oximetry

Pulse oximetry is used to assess the patient's arterial blood oxygen saturation. Without pulse oximetry, you may not notice the patient has a decreased arterial oxygen saturation of haemoglobin (SaO_2) until the saturation is between 80–85%. Pulse oximetry is simple to use, relatively cheap, non-invasive and provides an immediate, objective measure of arterial blood oxygen saturation. Oxygen saturation is a component of many physiological early warning systems (e.g. NEWS). All sick patients should have their oxygen saturation monitored (Chapter 2).

Principles of pulse oximetry

The pulse oximeter probe containing light-emitting diodes (LEDs) and a photoreceptor situated opposite, is placed across tissue, usually a finger or earlobe. Some of the light is transmitted through the tissues while some is absorbed. The ratio of transmitted to absorbed light is used to generate the peripheral arterial oxygen saturation (SpO_2) displayed as a digital reading, waveform, or both.

The displayed reading alters every 0.5–1 seconds, giving the average SpO_2 over the preceding 5–10 seconds.

Pulse oximeters have an audible tone related to the SpO_2 value, with a decreasing tone reflecting increasing hypoxaemia (unless the sound or alarm has been switched off). A poor signal can indicate a low blood pressure or poor tissue perfusion – reassess the patient.

Pulse oximeter readings must not be used in isolation – always look at the patient and clinical picture. Pulse oximetry measures only oxygen saturation, not content, and thus gives no indication of actual tissue oxygenation. Furthermore, the SpO_2 gives no information about adequate ventilation during oxygen therapy. A patient can be breathing inadequately and have a high carbon dioxide value despite a normal oxygen saturation. Arterial blood gas values are therefore needed in critically ill patients to assess oxygenation and ventilation.

Limitations of pulse oximetry

The relationship between oxygen saturation and arterial oxygen partial pressure (PaO_2) is demonstrated by the oxyhaemoglobin dissociation curve (Figure 9.1). The sinusoid shape of the curve means that an initial decrease from a normal PaO_2 is not accompanied by a decrease of similar magnitude in the oxygen saturation of the blood, and early hypoxaemia may be masked. At the point where the SpO_2 reaches 90–92%, the PaO_2 (see below) will have decreased from 12–14 kPa to 8 kPa. In other words, the amount of oxygen in the blood will be decreased by 25% for a fall of only 6–8% in SpO_2.

The output from a pulse oximeter relies on a comparison between current signal output and standardised reference data derived from healthy volunteers. Readings provided are thus limited by the scope of the population included in these studies, and become increasingly unreliable with increasing hypoxaemia. Below ~70% the displayed values are highly unreliable.

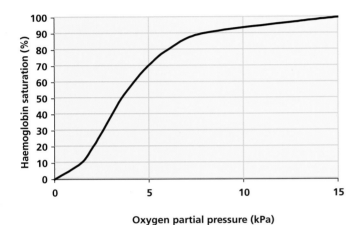

Figure 9.1 Haemoglobin oxygen dissociation curve

Errors with pulse oximetry can be caused by:

- Presence of other haemoglobins: carboxyhaemoglobin (carbon monoxide poisoning), methaemoglobin (congenital or acquired), fetal haemoglobins and sickling red cells (sickle cell disease).

- Surgical and imaging dyes (e.g. methylene blue) can cause falsely low saturation readings.

- Nail varnish (especially blue, black and green).

- High-ambient light levels (fluorescent and xenon lamps).

- Motion artefact.

- Reduced pulse volume:

  - hypotension

  - low cardiac output

  - vasoconstriction

  - hypothermia

Pulse oximeters are not affected by:

- Anaemia (reduced haemoglobin)

- Jaundice (hyperbilirubinaemia)

- Skin colour.

Pulse oximetry does not provide a reliable signal during CPR.

Uses of pulse oximetry

Pulse oximetry has four main uses:

1. detection of/screening for hypoxaemia

2. targeting oxygen therapy

3. routine monitoring (e.g. in high dependency settings)

4. diagnostic (e.g. sleep apnoea).

Targeted oxygen therapy

Give high-concentration oxygen immediately to critically ill patients with acute hypoxaemia (initial SpO_2 < 85%) or in the peri-arrest situation. Give this initially with an oxygen mask and reservoir ('non-rebreathing' mask) and an oxygen flow of 15 L min^{-1} (Figure 9.2). During cardiac arrest use 100% inspired oxygen concentration to maximise arterial oxygen content and delivery to the tissues.

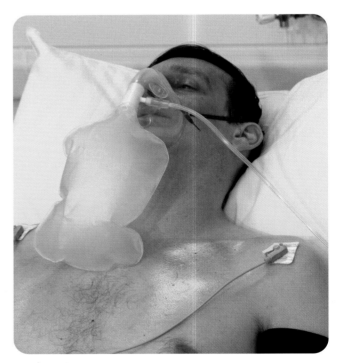

Figure 9.2 High-flow oxygen with a 'non-rebreathing' mask

If a return of spontaneous circulation (ROSC) has been achieved after cardiac arrest and the oxygen saturation of arterial blood can be monitored reliably with a pulse oximeter, adjust the inspired oxygen concentration to maintain a SpO_2 of 94–98%. If pulse oximetry (with a reliable reading) is unavailable, continue oxygen via a reservoir mask until definitive monitoring or assessment of oxygenation is available.

There is increasing evidence that a high blood oxygen concentration after cardiac arrest or a myocardial infarction can be harmful. There is much more evidence however, to say that too little oxygen is harmful and this is what we are trying to avoid by giving high-flow oxygen, and then adjusting it to achieve normal blood oxygen levels.

For example, in patients with a myocardial infarction or an acute coronary syndrome, aim to maintain an SpO_2 of 94–98%. This may be achievable without supplementary oxygen.

Special clinical situations

Patients with respiratory failure can be divided into two groups:

- Type I: low PaO_2 (< 8 kPa), normal $PaCO_2$ (< 7 kPa). In these patients it is safe to give a high concentration of oxygen initially with the aim of returning their PaO_2 to normal and then once clinically stable, adjusting the inspired oxygen concentration to maintain an SpO_2 of 94–98%.

- Type II: low PaO_2 (< 8 kPa), increased $PaCO_2$ (> 7 kPa). This is often described as hypercapnic respiratory failure and is often caused by COPD. If given excessive oxygen, these patients may develop worsening respiratory failure with further increases in $PaCO_2$ and the development of a respiratory acidosis. If unchecked, this will eventually lead to unconsciousness, and respiratory and cardiac arrest. **The target oxygen saturation in this at risk population is 88–92%.** However, when critically ill and their arterial blood oxygen saturation is unknown, give these patients high-flow oxygen initially; then analyse the arterial blood gases and use the results to adjust the inspired oxygen concentration. When clinically stable and a reliable pulse oximetry reading is obtained, adjust the inspired oxygen concentration to maintain an SpO_2 of 88–92%.

PaO_2 is partial pressure of oxygen which measures the amount of oxygen in arterial blood.

$PaCO_2$ is partial pressure of carbon dioxide which measures the amount of carbon dioxide in arterial blood . They are measured with a blood gas analyser.

Summary learning

- **Pulse oximetry enables arterial blood oxygen saturation to be monitored continuously.**
- **Use an inspired oxygen concentration of 100% until return of spontaneous circulation (ROSC) is achieved.**
- **After ROSC is achieved, and once the SpO_2 can be monitored reliably, titrate the inspired oxygen concentration to keep the SpO_2 in the range 94–98%.**

My key take-home messages from this chapter

Further reading

O'Driscoll BR, Howard LS, Davison AG. BTS guideline for emergency oxygen use in adult patients. Thorax 2008;63 Suppl 6:vi1-68.

Making decisions about CPR

Contents

- **The ethical principles that underpin decisions about CPR**
- **What constitutes good decision-making, effective communication and clear documentation of discussions and decisions**
- **Legal aspects of decisions about CPR**
- **When to withhold CPR**
- **When and when not to consider withdrawal of other treatments**

Learning outcomes

To enable you to:

- **Understand when it is and when it is not appropriate to attempt CPR**
- **Know when to stop CPR**
- **Consider the ethical and legal principles involved**
- **Consider who should make decisions about CPR**
- **Know what you and others should do to achieve good decisions about CPR**
- **Understand the importance of effective communication with all involved**
- **Understand the importance of effective documentation of decisions and discussions**

And to feel more confident in:

- **Making anticipatory decisions about CPR with your patients**
- **Encouraging others to follow best practice in decision-making**

Introduction

Although only a minority of people survives to make a complete recovery after receiving CPR, successful resuscitation attempts bring extended, precious life to many. If it is to be successful, CPR must be started without delay in those who may have a reversible cause for cardiac arrest. Used inappropriately – as with any treatment – CPR can do harm. When someone is dying from an irreversible cause, CPR is unlikely to work but can subject them to an undignified death, or even cause suffering and prolong the process of dying. Don't assume that everyone whose heart and breathing stop would consider survival a successful outcome. Prolonging life at all costs is not an appropriate goal of health care.

If a person is at risk of death or sudden cardiac arrest, consider in advance whether or not CPR could help them and whether they would want CPR. Whenever possible, make such advance plans as shared decisions with patients as part of a wider consideration of other care and realistic treatments that may or may not be appropriate for each individual.

ILS

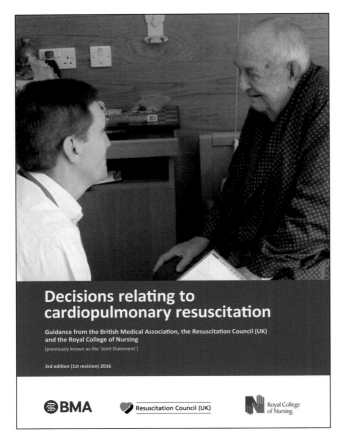

Figure 10.1 Decisions relating to cardiopulmonary resuscitation

Discuss advance decisions about CPR in the context of goals of care

Avoid focusing specifically on cardiac arrest or CPR or completing a form. Start by establishing a shared understanding of the patient's condition and likely future developments. Explore their priorities and preferences for their future care. Then discuss what types of care and realistic treatment will help them to achieve their goals of care, and whether or not they would want them, and explain relevant treatments that would not work for them or could do them harm. Discuss CPR within this context of their broader treatment options, which might include, for example, emergency admission to hospital, various types of organ support such as ventilation, or antibiotics for life-threatening infection.

Recording a person's wishes about these other aspects of their care and treatment, alongside recommendations about CPR, can help to guide immediate decision-making by health or care professionals faced with helping that person (who they may not have met before) in an emergency in which the patient has lost capacity to make or express decisions at the time.

Make sure that you are familiar with the approach and policy that is used in your health and care community or organisation. The Resuscitation Council (UK) has supported development of the ReSPECT process. For further information, see **www.respectprocess.org.uk**.

Principles

The four key principles of medical ethics are summarised in the box.

Autonomy requires people to be allowed and helped to make their own informed decisions, rather than having decisions made for them. A person with capacity must be adequately informed about the matter to be decided and free from undue pressure in making their decision. Autonomy allows an informed person to make a choice, even if that choice is considered illogical or incorrect by others, including health professionals.

Beneficence involves provision of benefit to an individual, while balancing benefit and risks. Commonly this will involve attempting CPR for cardiac arrest. If CPR will offer no benefit or the risks clearly outweigh any likely benefit it will mean withholding CPR. Beneficence includes also actions that benefit the wider community, such as providing a programme of public access defibrillation.

Non-maleficence means doing no harm. CPR should not be attempted in people in whom it will not succeed, where no benefit is likely but there will be a clear risk of doing harm.

Justice requires spreading benefits and risks equally within a society. If CPR is provided, it should be available to all who may benefit from it. There should be no discrimination purely on the grounds of factors such as age or disability. Justice does not imply an entitlement to expect or demand CPR for everyone. If limited resources are engaged in attempting CPR on people with no chance of benefit those resources may not be available when needed by others who are likely to benefit.

Detailed guidance, **Decisions relating to cardiopulmonary resuscitation**, has been published by the British Medical Association (BMA), Resuscitation Council (UK) (RC (UK)) and Royal College of Nursing (RCN) (Figure 10.1). It addresses ethical and legal aspects of decisions about CPR; the principles that underpin this guidance apply equally to the broader planning approach taken by the ReSPECT process and other treatment escalation plans. Laws relevant to CPR, including those on matters relating to capacity and consent, vary from nation to nation, both outside and within the UK.

Every decision about CPR must be based on a careful assessment of each individual's situation at any particular time. These decisions must never be dictated by 'blanket' policies. Individual decisions about CPR may be influenced by many factors, including personal beliefs and values, cultural or religious influences, ethical or legal considerations and social or economic circumstances.

Communication: discussing decisions about CPR with patients

Discussing decisions about CPR and other treatments that are seen as potentially life-sustaining can be challenging for patients, their families or carers and for health professionals. Many people welcome the opportunity to discuss their wishes, once they realise that the purpose is to plan with them what treatment would be best for them, not to deny them beneficial treatment. Specific skills training in having these sensitive conversations can help health professionals to communicate effectively and to recognise that these conversations are important and are not necessarily difficult. Explore your opportunities for such training as part of your professional development.

Don't force conversations on people who don't want them, but don't withhold them from those who do. Whenever possible, they should be undertaken by health professionals who know the person well, but that may not be possible when they are needed by someone with an acute illness or injury and no previous advance plan.

Effective communication is essential to ensure that decisions about treatments such as CPR are made well and understood clearly by all those involved. The courts have made clear that there should be a presumption in favour of involving patients in discussions about whether or not CPR will be attempted. This upholds the principle of autonomy and the provisions of the Human Rights Act (1998). If discussing a decision about CPR with a person is likely to cause them physical or psychological harm, such discussion may be omitted; the reasons for doing so should be documented clearly.

If a patient has capacity, discussions about CPR should usually involve shared decision-making, following the principles outlined in **Decisions relating to CPR** and in guidance from the General Medical Council. Requirements for effective communication include providing information in a format that the person can understand, and checking that they have understood it. They may need time and more than one discussion before they can reach a shared decision that they are comfortable with. They should be offered opportunities for further discussion and be made aware that they may change their decision if they wish to.

It is not necessary to discuss CPR with a patient if there is no reason to expect them to suffer cardiac arrest or die. However, if any patient wants to discuss CPR they must be given full opportunity to do so.

If the healthcare team is as certain as it can be that a person is dying as an inevitable result of underlying disease or a catastrophic health event, and that CPR would not re-start the heart and breathing for a sustained period, CPR should neither be offered nor attempted. Deciding to recommend that CPR is not attempted when it has no realistic prospect of success does not require the consent of the patient (or of those close to the patient). However, there is still a presumption in favour of informing a patient of such a decision and explaining the reasons for making it. A patient (or someone representing them) is not entitled to insist on receiving treatment that is clinically inappropriate. Health professionals are not obliged to offer or deliver treatment that they believe to be inappropriate. Explaining these matters requires sensitive discussion.

Communication: discussing decisions about CPR with those close to patients

Effective communication with those close to a patient (often but not always family members) and keeping them fully informed is an important component of high-quality health care. You must respect a patient's wishes regarding confidentiality, but most patients want family members or others close to them to be involved in discussions about treatments such as CPR and to have their support in making these decisions.

You must use discussion with those close to a patient to guide any decision made in the best interests of a person who lacks capacity. Explore what the patient would have wanted and what would be in their best interests (rather than what the family or carers may want). Those close to the patient must not be burdened with feeling that they are being asked to make a decision about CPR as this responsibility rests with the senior clinician.

Communication: discussing decisions about CPR when a patient lacks capacity

If a person lacks capacity, they can still be involved in decision-making to the limit of their ability. Formal assessment of their capacity should be undertaken and recorded. Decisions about their treatment, including about CPR, must be made in their best interests. If (as defined in the Mental Capacity Act 2005 (MCA 2005) – which applies in England & Wales) they have made a valid and applicable Advance Decision to Refuse Treatment (ADRT) that refuses CPR "even if their life is at risk" that ADRT is legally binding and must be respected. If a person who lacks capacity has a legal proxy (e.g. a 'welfare attorney') with power to make such decisions on their behalf, that person must be involved in the decision-making process. The courts have stated also that, when considering a decision about CPR for a person who lacks capacity, there is a duty to consult anyone engaged in caring for them or interested in their welfare. In some circumstances the law requires you to involve others. For example, the MCA 2005 requires an Independent Mental Capacity Advocate (IMCA) to speak on behalf of a person who lacks capacity and has no other representatives, guiding a best-interests decision by the senior clinician.

However, if a person is critically ill and an urgent decision is needed in order to plan the best care for them, that decision should not be delayed if their family or other carers cannot be contacted, or there is not enough time to appoint or contact an IMCA. Make the decision that is in the person's best interests, but also make and record a clear plan to consult their family or others close to them, or to contact an IMCA, at the earliest practicable opportunity. Document the basis for any decision clearly and fully.

Deciding whether or not to attempt CPR

Whether or not to attempt CPR at the time of a cardiac arrest requires immediate decision by the person or persons present. That decision will be influenced by their role, training and experience, as well as by the immediate circumstances. Where a recommendation has been considered and recorded in advance it can help those present at the moment of crisis to make the best possible immediate decision (see below). The same applies to other types of emergency care or treatment that may be considered in an emergency in which the person does not have capacity to make and express choices.

The overall responsibility for proper decision-making and planning about CPR, rests with the senior health professional in charge of the person's care at the time. When making advance plans there should be appropriate consultation with other health professionals involved, as well as appropriate discussion with the person themselves and those close to them.

If a difference of opinion arises between the healthcare team and the patient or their representatives this can usually be resolved by careful discussion and explanation. If not, a second clinical opinion should be offered. Seeking a decision by legal authorities may involve delay and uncertainty. Formal legal judgement may be needed if there are irreconcilable differences between the parties. In difficult cases, the senior clinician may wish to seek legal advice from his/her indemnity provider or other professional organisation.

Recording advance plans about CPR

Make sure that any recommendation on whether or not to attempt CPR and the reasons for that recommendation are documented clearly and that (as far as is reasonably possible) the record is available immediately if it is needed in a crisis. For example, if such a recommendation is recorded on a paper form, this should be readily available to help an ambulance clinician decide whether to attempt CPR in a person's home. People should be encouraged and helped to make those close to them aware of their wishes and resulting recommendations, and of where to find the record of these.

It has been common practice to record only DNACPR 'decisions', using a specific 'DNACPR form'. However, anticipatory recommendations about CPR are best made in the context of other care and treatment choices, and it is important to record recommendations to attempt CPR as well as recommendations not to do so. Don't assume that people at risk of cardiac arrest or death would all want to receive CPR; whenever possible offer people the chance to plan ahead, and to make an informed choice.

Various forms have been developed in different places to record people's treatment decisions in advance. The RC (UK) favours the use of a standard document that is used and accepted by all health and care provider organisations, so that it is effective across geographical and organisational boundaries. It supports use of the ReSPECT process and form: www.respectprocess.org.uk.

As an ILS provider, try to ensure that decisions about CPR are recorded fully, clearly and accurately. Make sure also that you understand the status of any such document. Most such forms are not legally binding and are intended to guide immediate clinical decision-making by those present at a moment of crisis. It would be unwise to ignore such a document that records an agreed or shared decision and/or the person's express wishes. However, if you encounter an arrest in circumstances that you believe were not those envisaged when the decision was recorded it may be appropriate to attempt CPR (e.g. to relieve choking or a blocked tracheostomy tube).

Some recorded advance decisions are legally binding, such as an ADRT (see above). If a person with capacity has recorded refusal of CPR in an ADRT you must respect this, provided the document is valid and that the immediate circumstances are those that were envisaged when the ADRT was recorded. Whilst the MCA 2005 requires an ADRT to be in writing, signed and witnessed, a refusal of treatment does not have to be in writing in order to be valid. If an informed person has expressed clear and consistent refusal verbally, this is likely to have the same status as a written advance refusal.

The term 'advance statement' may apply to any expression of preferences by a patient. Occasionally people have taken the more extreme step of having a DNACPR instruction tattooed on their chest. This is not considered a legally binding refusal; its expression of their wishes at the time must be balanced against the possibility that they may not have been fully informed, that they may have since changed their mind, or that the current circumstances are not those that they had envisaged when the tattoo was created.

Where no explicit advance decision has been made and the express wishes of the patient are unknown there is a presumption that health professionals will make all reasonable and appropriate efforts to resuscitate someone from cardiac arrest. In sudden out-of-hospital cardiac arrest, those present may not know the victim's situation or wishes. Even if an ADRT has been recorded, it may not be available. In these circumstances CPR can be started immediately and further information obtained when possible. There is no ethical difficulty in stopping a resuscitation attempt if the health professionals performing CPR are then presented with a valid, recorded ADRT refusing CPR or a valid DNACPR decision.

Communicating recommendations to health and care teams

Good communication within the team is an essential component of high-quality, safe health care. When an advance recommendation is made about whether or not to attempt CPR it should be communicated clearly to all those who may need to know about it and act on it.

The basis for the recommendation, details of those involved in making it, and details of discussions with patients and those close to them should be recorded. The recommendation itself should be recorded in a way that is immediately accessible and recognisable by those present, should the patient suffer cardiac arrest.

There should be effective verbal communication with all those caring for the person and robust written and/or electronic documentation to ensure that recommendations are known about and the records remain available if the person travels to a different location, however briefly. Within a hospital, that might involve, for example, attending a radiology or physiotherapy department for investigation or treatment. In the community, it might involve, for example, attending a healthcare appointment or going out with or visiting friends or family.

When to withhold CPR

When an informed person with capacity refuses CPR as a potential treatment option it should be withheld. If CPR would not re-start the heart and breathing for a sustained period because a person is dying as an inevitable result of underlying disease or a catastrophic health event CPR should be withheld. Although these statements seem relatively straightforward, people may interpret them in different ways. In particular, what constitutes 'futility' in relation to CPR, what constitutes 'successful resuscitation' and what constitutes 'a sustained period' may be viewed differently by individual patients and by individual health professionals.

Many out-of-hospital cardiac arrests are attended by emergency medical technicians or paramedics, who face dilemmas about when CPR will not succeed and when it should be stopped. In general, CPR will be started in out-of-hospital cardiac arrest unless there is a valid ADRT refusing it or a record of a valid DNACPR decision. Ambulance service guidelines allow trained personnel to refrain from starting CPR in defined situations, for example in people with mortal injuries such as decapitation or hemicorporectomy, incineration, rigor mortis and hypostasis. In such cases, the ambulance clinician may identify that death has occurred but cannot certify the cause of death (which in most countries can be done only by a doctor or coroner).

Similar recognition that death has occurred and is irreversible and a resulting decision not to start CPR may be made by experienced nurses working in the community or in settings that provide care for people who are terminally or chronically ill. Whenever possible, advance recommendations about CPR should be considered as part of advance care planning before they are needed in a crisis.

A recorded DNACPR recommendation means that it is not appropriate to start CPR for cardiorespiratory arrest, unless the circumstances of the arrest are not those envisaged when the recommendation was recorded. Make sure that all other care is given in accordance with the person's treatment plan and is of the highest standard. This may include elements of care such as giving nutrition or

recording physiological observations, and treatments such as pain relief or sedation. As an ILS provider, make sure that a properly made and recorded DNACPR recommendation does not (through your actions or those of others) lead to withholding from a patient of other care or treatment.

Decisions about implanted cardioverter-defibrillators

When a person who is approaching the end of their life has an implanted cardioverter-defibrillator (ICD), a discussion with them about CPR should prompt also a sensitive discussion about whether and when they may wish to have the shock function of their ICD deactivated. A proportion of people who die with an active ICD in place will receive shocks from the device in the last hours or days of their life. These are usually painful and can be distressing for the patient and for those close to them.

However, it must not be assumed that a DNACPR decision automatically warrants deactivation of an ICD. Some people may wish to have prompt treatment from an ICD, but choose not to have CPR for cardiac arrest, which is much more traumatic, would have a lower chance of success and greater risk of harm. Detailed guidance on this topic has been published by the Resuscitation Council (UK), British Cardiovascular Society and National Council for Palliative Care, together with a short clinical guide and an information leaflet for patients.

Defining 'success' and 'futility'

Achieving return of spontaneous circulation (ROSC) does not mean that CPR has been successful. A resuscitation attempt can only be regarded as successful if it restores a patient to a duration and quality of life that they themselves regard as worth having. Attempted resuscitation can only be regarded as being truly futile if it has no chance of achieving that outcome. These statements emphasise the importance, whenever possible, of knowing a person's wishes and beliefs in advance.

Predicting outcome

Predicting the outcome from CPR for cardiac arrest is far from easy. The outcome is dependent on many factors, including the prior state of health of the patient and the times from arrest to starting CPR and from arrest to defibrillation. Predictors of non-survival after attempted resuscitation have been published, but do not have sufficient predictive value to be used in clinical practice in the immediate period after ROSC.

Avoiding discrimination

Inevitably, clinical judgements have to be made. There will be uncertainties when decisions are needed for patients with conditions such as heart failure, chronic respiratory disease, asphyxia, major trauma, head injury and neurological disease. It is crucial that decisions are non-discriminatory and, for example, do not deprive people of CPR purely on the grounds of factors such as age or a disability. The age of the patient may be considered in the decision-making process but is only a relatively weak independent predictor of outcome. However, many elderly people have significant comorbidity, which influences outcome.

Remember also to avoid discriminating by attempting CPR with no realistic chance of benefit on a patient, simply because they are younger or because of an assumption that they would want this.

Summary learning

- **In the event of cardiac arrest, attempt CPR immediately and effectively unless there is a clear reason to withhold it.**

- **Whenever possible, anticipatory decisions about CPR are best made early (rather than at a time of crisis) and in the context of other choices about a person's care and treatment.**

- **Good communication is essential to ensure that anticipatory decisions about CPR are made well and understood clearly by all those involved.**

- **There should be a presumption in favour of involving patients in discussions about whether or not CPR will be attempted, but there is no requirement to offer to attempt CPR when it will not succeed.**

- **Communicate effectively and sensitively about CPR with patients and with those close to patients.**

- **Communicate recommendations about CPR effectively to all health and care professionals involved.**

- **If a valid ADRT refusing CPR has been made this is legally binding; do not attempt CPR unless the circumstances of the arrest are not those envisaged when the ADRT was made.**

- **If a valid DNACPR decision has been recorded do not attempt CPR unless the circumstances of the arrest are not those envisaged when the decision was made.**

- **If CPR will not re-start the heart and breathing do not start CPR.**

- **If continuing CPR will not be successful make the decision to stop.**

- **Record anticipatory decisions about CPR carefully and try to ensure that the record will available when needed.**

- **Do not allow a DNACPR decision to deprive a patient from receiving any other appropriate care or treatment.**

My key take-home messages from this chapter

Further reading

British Medical Association, Resuscitation Council (UK) and Royal College of Nursing. Decisions relating to cardiopulmonary resuscitation. 3rd Edition, First revision 2016.
https://www.resus.org.uk/dnacpr/decisions-relating-to-cpr/

General Medical Council. Treatment and care towards the end of life. 2010.
www.gmc-uk.org

Pitcher D, Fritz Z, Wang M, Spiller, J. Emergency care and resuscitation plans. BMJ 2017;356:j876.

Resuscitation Council (UK). British Cardiovascular Society and National Council for Palliative Care. Deactivation of implantable cardioverter-defibrillators towards the end of life.
https://www.resus.org.uk/publications/cardiovascular-implanted-electronic-devices/

The Scottish Government. Adults with Incapacity (Scotland) Act 2000: A short guide to the Act.
www.gov.scot/Topics/Justice/law/awi/010408awiwebpubs/infopublications

UK Government. Mental Capacity Act 2005 Code of Practice.
https://www.gov.uk/government/collections/mental-capacity-act-makingdecisions

Drugs commonly used during the treatment of cardiac arrest

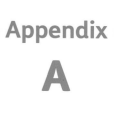

Drug	Shockable (VF/pVT)	Non-shockable (PEA/Asystole)
ADRENALINE	• Dose: 1 mg (10 mL 1:10,000 or 1 mL 1:1,000) IV • Given after the third shock once compressions have been resumed • Repeated every 3–5 minutes (alternate loops) • Give without interrupting chest compressions	• Dose: 1 mg (10 mL 1:10,000 or 1 mL 1:1,000) IV • Given as soon as circulatory access is obtained • Repeated every 3–5 minutes (alternate loops) • Give without interrupting chest compressions
	Adrenaline has been the primary sympathomimetic drug for the management of cardiac arrest for 45 years. Its alpha-adrenergic effects cause systemic vasoconstriction, which increases coronary and cerebral perfusion pressures. The beta-adrenergic actions of adrenaline (inotropic, chronotropic) may increase coronary and cerebral blood flow, but concomitant increases in myocardial oxygen consumption and ectopic ventricular arrhythmias (particularly in the presence of acidaemia), transient hypoxaemia because of pulmonary arteriovenous shunting, impaired microcirculation, and increased post cardiac arrest myocardial dysfunction may offset these benefits. Although there is no evidence of long-term benefit from the use of adrenaline, the improved short-term survival documented in some studies warrants its continued use pending the outcome of ongoing clinical trials.	
AMIODARONE	• Dose: 300 mg bolus IV diluted in 5% dextrose (or other suitable solvent) to a volume of 20 mL • Given during chest compressions after three defibrillation attempts • Further dose of 150 mg if VF/pVT persists after five defibrillation attempts	• Not indicated for PEA or asystole
	Amiodarone is a membrane-stabilising anti-arrhythmic drug that increases the duration of the action potential and refractory period in atrial and ventricular myocardium. Atrioventricular conduction is slowed, and a similar effect is seen with accessory pathways. Amiodarone has a mild negative inotropic action and causes peripheral vasodilation through non-competitive alpha-blocking effects. Although there is no evidence of long-term benefit from the use of amiodarone, it may improve short-term survival warranting its continued use pending the outcome of ongoing clinical trials. Amiodarone should be flushed with 0.9% sodium chloride or 5% dextrose. When amiodarone is unavailable, consider an initial dose of 100 mg (1–1.5 mg kg^{-1}) of lidocaine for VF/pVT refractory to three shocks. Give an additional bolus of 50 mg if necessary. The total dose should not exceed 3 mg kg^{-1} during the first hour.	
FLUIDS	Infuse fluids rapidly if hypovolaemia is suspected. Use 0.9% sodium chloride. Hartmann's solution or PlasmaLyte, or blood for major haemorrhage. Avoid dextrose, which is redistributed away from the intravascular space rapidly and causes hyperglycaemia, which may worsen neurological outcome and survival after cardiac arrest.	

ILS

www.resus.org.uk	Resuscitation Council (UK)
www.erc.edu	European Resuscitation Council
www.ilcor.org	International Liaison Committee on Resuscitation
www.americanheart.org	American Heart Association
www.nice.org.uk	The National Institute for Health and Care Excellence (NICE)
www.bhf.org.uk	British Heart Foundation
www.ics.ac.uk	Intensive Care Society
www.aagbi.org	Association of Anaesthetists of Great Britain and Ireland
www.bestbets.org	Best evidence topics in emergency medicine
www.bcs.com	British Cardiac Society
www.escardio.org	European Society of Cardiology
www.esicm.org	European Society of Intensive Care Medicine

 Resuscitation Guidelines   Resuscitation Council (UK) courses

 iResus app – easy access to the Resuscitation Guidelines

 Lifesaver app – a new way to learn CPR

 @ResusCouncilUK   Resuscitation Council UK   ResusCouncilUK

ILS